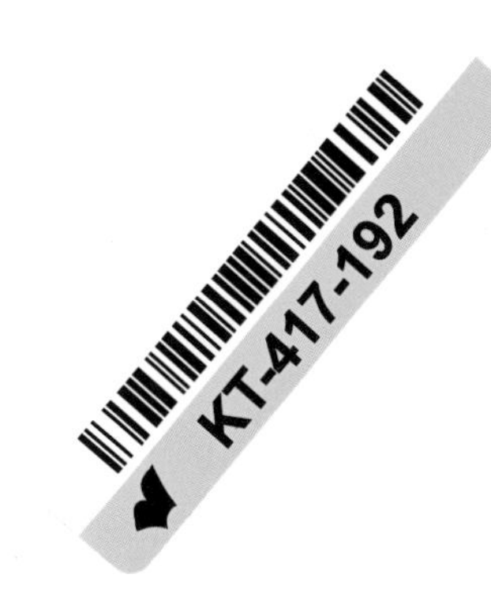

Intermediate Care

Models in Practice

Barbara Vaughan MSc RGN
Judith Lathlean DPhil

Published by
King's Fund Publishing
11-13 Cavendish Square
London W1G 0AN

ISBN 1 85717 273 6

A CIP catalogue record of this book is available from the British Library.

Further copies of this book can be obtained from the King's Fund bookshop telephone 020 7307 2591.

This report has been produced to promote good practice and quality improvement in health and social care. It has not been professionally copy-edited or proof-read.

Table of Contents

Acknowledgements

This report could not have been prepared without the help and support we have received from colleagues in both operational and strategic roles who are developing a range of Intermediate Care services. The innovations are too great in number to all be included within this text. Nevertheless, the willingness of many people to share information in relation to both the service developments and the complex processes of implementation have all added to the manner in which this report has been developed.

We are also grateful to the Department of Health who have not only funded this project but given support, advice and practical help throughout the production time of the report. Their contribution in providing related information and constructive criticism has been highly valued.

A final word of thanks to the project steering group who have also provided that essential support and advise which underpins work of this nature.

Part One

Introduction

There has, over the past few years, been a growing interest in the introduction of Intermediate Care services with a primary function of supporting people in the transition between acute, primary and social care. There remains, however, lack of consensus about the nature of these services, the manner in which they should be developed, and whether they should substitute for, or be additional to, more traditional options. Relatively little attention has been paid to their development to date and where initiatives have flourished they has largely been dependant on the drive of individuals, rather than as part of a wider strategic initiative.

The purpose of this publication is to address some of these issues. The intention is not to offer a blue print for future development of Intermediate Care but to share information about current practice initiatives. To this end a range of different models have been described in a variety of different care settings and short and long term implications have been presented for debate.

Background

Defining intermediate care

As interest in Intermediate Care has grown it has rapidly become apparent that there is a fundamental lack of conceptual clarity about the subject under debate. While it can be argued that in defining a subject too tightly some of the creativity of development may be lost, without a common understanding of what is meant by Intermediate Care, it is not possible to either explore its introduction at an operational or strategic level or to evaluate its efficacy. To this end a tight working definition was initially developed which suggested that Intermediate Care encompassed:

> *That range of services designed to facilitate the transition from hospital to home, and from medical dependence to functional independence, where the objectives of care are not primarily medical, the patient's discharge destination is anticipated, and a clinical outcome of recovery (or restoration of health) is desired.*[1]

Over time, and with practical experience, this original definition has been broadened to encompass:

> *Those services which will help to divert admission to an acute care setting through timely therapeutic interventions which aim to divert a physiological crisis or offer recuperative services at or near a person's own home.*

---

[1] Steiner A (1997) *Intermediate Care: A conceptual framework and review of the literature* London King's Fund

Intermediate Care – what it is not

The clear focus which Intermediate Care has on health gain differentiates it from:

- convalescence – which allows time for people to heal but has no active therapeutic input
- hotel beds – which bring people near services but offer no therapy
- long stay beds – where it is unlikely that there will be sufficient recovery for people to regain independent living
- movement of services – from one setting to another e.g. the shift in treatment of deep vein thrombosis from acute to primary care
- another layer in the service – rather it is being developed in response to what has become known as the 'black hole', where no targeted services have been available to help the transition between acute, primary and social care[2].

Thus Intermediate Care is one of a continuum of services which bridge between social, primary and acute care but with a clear, separate focus. While the majority of Intermediate Care services are used by older people, many other patients groups including children and people with ongoing disabilities can gain benefit.

Why now?

While the manner in which Intermediate Care is described offers no surprises it does present a considerable challenge to those involved in its implementation. There are, however, a range of contextual factors which appear to be influencing the growing interest.

Firstly there has been increasing pressure on the acute sector, exacerbated by multiple factors including winter pressures, increasing medical admissions, and technical and pharmacological developments. These pressures can be illustrated by a review of changes in terms of bed numbers, admissions and length of stay over the last twenty years.

Acute and geriatric beds – In the twenty years up to 1997/98 acute beds fell from 155,000 to 108,000. During the same period geriatric beds fell from 56,000 to 30,000. Since 1970 the number of beds in the acute, geriatric and maternity specialties has fallen from 240,000 to 150,000.

Admissions – During the twenty years up to 1997/98 general and acute[3] ordinary admissions (finished consultant episodes) increased from 4.560m to 6.514m – that is at a rate of 1.8% a year. Since 1975, ordinary general and acute admission rates per thousand population have increased by an average of 3.5% a year for those aged 65 and over. This compares to 1.6% for all ages.

---

[2] Vaughan B, Steiner A, Hanford L (1999) *The Shape of the Team* London King's Fund

[3] General and acute is defined as acute plus geriatric (excluding well babies)

Length of stay – From 1981 to 1996/97 average acute length of stay (per finished consultant episode) decreased from 9.3 to 5.0 days while average geriatric length of stay decreased from 66.1 to 18.6 days.

In summary while there are fewer beds available more people are receiving care for shorter periods of time.

Secondly we have an ageing population. To illustrate this, the Personal Social Services Research Unit, in a recent report on demand for long term care for elderly people, projected continued growth in the numbers of elderly people[4]. They predicted that the number of people in England aged 65 and over would rise by almost 57% between 1995 and 2031, and the number of people over 85 years of age would rise by 79% over the same period.

Thirdly, there is a growing suggestion that some people in acute care settings are being inappropriately placed[5,6]. The 1998 Report of the Emergency Services Action Team (ESAT) questioned whether older people are being moved into long stay care prematurely. They noted that older patients experiencing an acute episode undergo complex changes in their dependency levels very quickly. A decision to place them in long term care at the end of an in-patient stay may no longer be valid two or three weeks later as the patient begins to recover former levels of independence. ESAT concluded that this pointed strongly to the need to invest in proven forms of Intermediate Care and rehabilitation which have been assessed for their clinical and cost-effectiveness, and which can equip patients to return home.

In addition policy changes are placing greater emphasis on community care with delivery of services closer to people's homes. A shared concern that there should be equity of access to the right care in the right place at the right time is leading to widespread debate about current geographical variations in service provision and a need for more effective sharing of models of good practice, especially as they relate to care in the community. There is, however, also concern that there should not be repetition of the difficulties faced with the decentralisation of mental health services a decade ago, without assurance that there is a sufficiently strong community based infrastructure to support the devolution of some services.

Pressures on social services and delays in hospital discharge, as both funds and availability of places are stretched, has also led to exploratory partnerships between health and social services, a move which is now supported through policy[7]. While the adage of troubles shared being troubles

---

[4] Personal Social Services Research Unit (1998) *Demand for long-term care: projections of long-term care finance for elderly people* London School of Economics

[5] Audit Commission (1992) *Lying in Wait: the use of medical beds in acute hospitals* London HMSO

[6] Evans A, Griffiths P (1994) *The Development of a Nursing-led In-patient Service* London King's Fund

[7] Department of Health (1998) *Partnership in Action: New Opportunities for Joint Working Between Health and Social Services* London DoH

halved may not be entirely fulfilled in this instance there is no doubt of the success of some of the health and social service partnerships which can act as models for future development.[8]

Triggers and barriers to action

It should be stressed that the concept of Intermediate Care services is not new. Both the patient population and the type of service can be easily recognised by those involved. The question then is 'Why – if the need is so familiar – have Intermediate Care services not been explored, developed or evaluated more fully in the past?' Debates around this question raise several issues of note, mainly concerned with the manner in which the services cross traditional professional and organisational boundaries.

One concern, in a resource limited health service, is that any new development, once it goes beyond pilot stage, must have substitution implications. Thus if Intermediate Care services are to be developed on a large scale it must be at a cost to another area of service delivery. Yet there are suggestions that the economic efficacy of Intermediate Care cannot be felt through a small pilot study which does not have an economy of scale[9]. Hence a dilemma occurs. For the full impact to be felt there is a need to increase the scale of Intermediate Care services but this, in turn, may meet resistance as it would necessitate a reduction elsewhere in service provision. That such obstacles can be overcome is evident by the number of inclusions in this publication. Nevertheless they can act as a significant barrier to development.

A second issue is lack of awareness, both inter- and intra-professionally, of the level of service which can be provided in settings, and by teams, other than that with which the practitioner is familiar[10]. Thus the manner in which services are currently configured, with clear boundaries between acute, primary and social care, mitigates a further disincentive, as does the segregated way in which professional education is offered. Such situations can be further exacerbated by lack of coterminous boundaries between different service sectors, difficulty in developing multi-agency work and in pooling budgets to a common purpose.

A third concern to date has been around evidence of the clinical and economic efficacy of Intermediate Care services. They are notoriously difficult to evaluate, partly because of the fluid nature of their development and the difficulty in identifying true comparators, but also because the indicators of success are not easily subject to direct or quasi-measurement. Hence in an environment which is rightly driven by concern about evidence based practice, the nature of evidence in relation to Intermediate Care is, to date, often small scale and qualitative. For example in exploring the value of Hospital at Home schemes only five reports match the rigorous Cochrane

---

[8] Younger-Ross S, Lomax T (1998) Outlands: Five Years on *Managing Community Care* Vol 6 Issue 1 37-40

[9] Steiner A, Vaughan B, Hanford L (1999) *Intermediate Care: Shifting the Money* London King's Fund

[10] Vaughan B, Steiner A, Handford L (1999) *Intermediate Care: The Shape of the Team* London King's Fund

criteria[11] despite a much wider number of studies being available in the literature. While there is an urgent need for further research, data to date provides the opportunity for conceptual rather than statistical assurance.

The time for change

Within this context it is evident that the time is ripe for change. There is, however, less clarity about what shape that change should take and what time scale should be followed. There is a needs driven thrust to explore alternative options at both an operational and a strategic level and there are many examples where the origins of new developments can be traced to either source, sometimes, but not always in synchrony. That whole systems approaches are of value is widely acknowledged but while there are some excellent examples of such practice they remain the exception rather than the rule.

Structure of this publication

The remainder of this report has been divided into four distinct sections, each of which can stand alone or be accessed as part of the whole document, according to the interest and need of the reader. An introduction to each section is given below in order to help people to access those parts which relate most closely to their interests.

Part two – models in practice

In this section short descriptions have been included of seven different approaches to service development under the broad definition of Intermediate Care. The inclusions have been selected because each one offers a different approach to a common concern, rather than because each one is either unique or a 'best' single solution. Recognition has been given to the many contextual factors which have influenced selection at a local level. Thus, while each of the initiatives was driven by the shared concerns of excessive pressure on acute and social care beds, and for the development of services which were specifically focused on the needs of patients in transition, the solutions offered vary considerably.

Common features are that the services have been established for more than two years and the provision is likely to be sustained; that funding arrangements are explicit; that there is some form of evaluation, albeit still in the early phases and that those involved are willing to share their experiences of both successes and difficulties. Examples have been included where the drive has come from social services, primary care or acute care, with both provider and commissioner

---

[11] Sheppard S, Lliffe S (1999) *Effectiveness of hospital at home compared to in-patient hospital care* (Cochrane review) in: The Cochrane Library, Issue 1 Oxford: Update Software

involvement, thus highlighting the range of issues which have led to their introduction. Finally, in each instance one or more contact names have been included to assist in sharing and networking.

Part three – developing a strategy

In this section two different examples have been included which describe the way in which a provider unit and a commissioning unit have set about exploring an agenda for future provision, offering an overview of their longer term strategic plans. Tools which have been developed to explore local need are discussed, alongside the manner in which alternative options were investigated and encompassed into local plans.

In neither case are these examples included as a blue print for the future but as a stimulus for debate and as exemplars on which others can build.

Part four – introducing Intermediate Care: short and long term issues for debate

In part four of the report some of the recurring themes which have arisen in relation to the development of Intermediate Care services are explored. Both drivers and inhibitors from the examples included in previous sections have been collated in this concluding chapter in order to preserve some anonymity for the contributors.

In addition wider implications for the shape of future services, professional education, cross boundary work for organisations and individuals, research and budgetary considerations are raised as part of the potential long term agenda for the development of health and social care.

Part five – a directory of development in Intermediate Care

The final part of this report contains brief details of a further 71 sites which have been involved in similar initiatives to the ones described earlier in the text. Each contributor has provided a summary of the services which they have developed at the acute, primary and social care interface and given contact details to facilitate wider networking. Space has limited the number of entries which it has been possible to include. Hence clinical diversity has been the deciding factor in the entries presented here. This directory is seen as a starting point to which additional local and national information can be added over time.

Part Two

The models described in this section have each been developed from a different perspective. They have been included in order to demonstrate variations in the way in which the interface between acute, primary and social care has been addressed in different settings and by different organisations.

The models included are:

- a GP led primary care directorate within an acute DGH
- a primary care led rapid response scheme
- a consultant led service within acute care providing a link between acute and primary services
- a nurse-led in-patient facility in acute care
- a nurse-led service in a community hospital
- a residential rehabilitation service managed by social services
- a combined Trust offering a range of intermediate care services for children

Each of the services is continuously evolving and developing with time. Some have already moved on from the descriptions included here in response to need, experience and increased competence and confidence.

Ealing Hospital NHS Trust

Ealing Intermediate Care Service

Purpose of the service

The Ealing Intermediate Care Service (ICS) has been developed following the success of the Winter Pressure and Challenge Fund projects in 1996/7, with Ealing health, social care and voluntary agencies joining forces to provide a comprehensive combination of Intermediate Care services. These "seek to maintain adults at home safely, in health and as independently as possible, by preventing inappropriate admission and by facilitating prompt discharge".[12]

Context

As with so many other places, Ealing has, over the past few years, faced increasing pressure in both health and social services. While the local elderly population is relatively stable in number, and predicted to stay that way, there had been a steady increase in emergency admissions of older people during the winter months (Figure one). In addition, there was an increasingly high demand for residential and nursing home care, with more than 60 people in March 1997 waiting for social support in order to return home from hospital. General practitioners were dissatisfied with services, social services could not respond to demand and the pressure on acute beds was becoming intolerable.

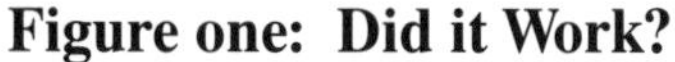

Figure one: Did it Work?

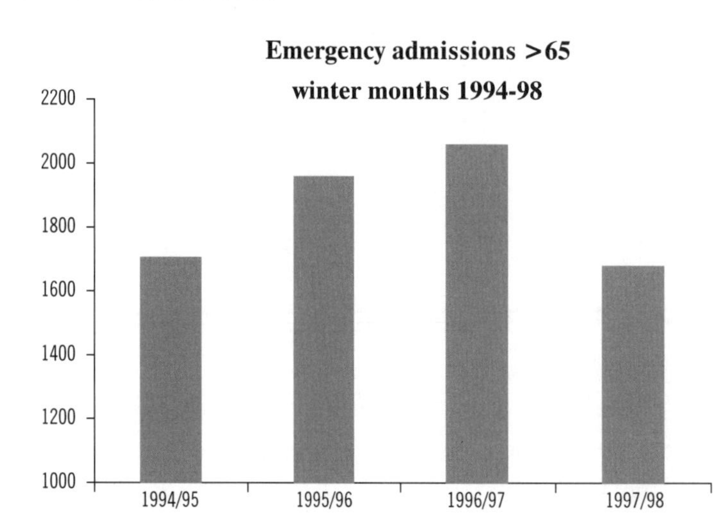

[12] Ealing Intermediate Care Services Information Pack

It was against this background that representatives from the three sectors (acute, primary and social care), in conjunction with voluntary organisations, joined forces to plan a way forward, taking a whole systems approach. Each of the managers was new in post and aware that something had to change. They were willing to take reasonable risk and to compromise when necessary in order to develop services in response to need.

Getting going

The collaborative nature of the Ealing scheme offered the opportunity for a range of different initiatives to be introduced over the winter of 1997/8 in order to reduce the impact of winter pressures. CATS (Community Assessment Team) in A&E - was the overall term for community services that were provided initially, which encompassed the support of an Occupational Therapist and the Rapid Response team (see below). As the services have expanded, co-ordination of the whole Intermediate Care initiative has been managed through the development of an independent directorate within the acute trust. It is led by a general practitioner who has brought together and rationalised the range of services which had been offered through acute and primary care, social services and the voluntary sector. These services now encompass:

Admission avoidance in A and E – this function is concerned with preventing unnecessary admission or aiding patient transfer to mainstream services and is managed by a Core Assessment Team (see below). It is offered to the mainly 65+ age group who may be referred from either acute or primary care, but the greatest number is identified in the Accident and Emergency department. Holistic multi-disciplinary assessment is available leading to:

- 'major packages of care' which encompass both social and rehabilitative support and are seen as admission avoidance strategies, therefore saving bed days
- 'minor packages' which aim to avoid readmission or the 'revolving door syndrome' by providing advice, therapy equipment or referral to an alternative source of help.

Between 45 and 65 people are offered care at any one time with a roughly equal distribution between major and minor packages. Minor care can, on the whole, be slotted in between other work. Hence the major financial demand relates to delivery of major packages of care.

Post Discharge Rehab – this aims to increase independence for the recipient, thereby reducing long term demand on Social Care. A package of intensive domiciliary therapy and home-care is planned for adult, medically stable patients so that they can benefit from early discharge from the acute trust. Care can be given for a period of up to six weeks. The people offering this service have now been assimilated into the Core Assessment Team.

Post discharge monitoring – this service is offered to help support older people who may have difficulty in coping after discharge, through the provision of post discharge telephone monitoring. If a difficulty is reported, a home assessment and package of care can be activated, or referral made to another agency e.g. voluntary sector.

Step Down Services – these provide early discharge to a residential or nursing home bed (whichever the patient needs) for patients who are awaiting long term placement, who no longer need acute medical care but who have not yet been allocated mainstream funding. By early placement of the patients in appropriate settings, acute beds are released.

Respite Care – as part of the overall Intermediate Care service respite care can be offered in either residential or nursing home facilities. The aim here is to avoid unnecessary admission, and to provide full care and rehabilitation for a short period

Red Cross – Home from Hospital – this service aims to assist in the smooth transition between hospital and home, providing volunteer escorts on discharge from A&E or wards, and short term home support. There are around 40 volunteers involved with the scheme, who provide a 'settling in service' for between 30 and 40 people a month. The possibility of expanding to cover other areas of care is currently being explored. The volunteers also assist in A&E at lunchtime, and in the Trust's discharge lounge.

Age Concern – COPE is an at risk register of vulnerable people, coupled with a weekly monitoring phone call by volunteers. They also offer Fallsafe, which has a team of trained volunteers who undertake risk assessment in the home and provide a 'handyman' to undertake minor repairs.

Staffing and support

Ealing believes that the time has passed for running pilot schemes and they now have a clinical directorate with specific responsibility for all intermediate care services, set up in June 1998. The team is led by a clinical director with a background in general practice, supported by a service manager who is a social worker. Several early initiatives have been encompassed into the current *Core Assessment Team* which includes:

District nurse	1
Social Worker	2.5
Occupational therapist	3
Physiotherapist	2
Therapy assistant	1
Administrator	0.5

Other members of the directorate include:

Respiratory nurse	1
Discharge Liaison Team	
District nurse	2
Placement officer	1
Administrator	1

Telephone monitoring
Community nurses 1.8

In addition there is a service evaluator and an NHS management trainee as part of the overall directorate. The team are supported by voluntary organisations (Red Cross and Age Concern) who receive some financial assistance to off-set their running costs.

Active attention has been paid to the learning needs of the team on two fronts. Training consultants have been used to help develop the cohesion of the team in order to ensure clear patterns of communication and good working relations. In addition there is an 'in house' programme of 'cross skilling'. This programme is needs driven, and based on the premise that any member of the core assessment team can ensure an initial holistic assessment for the patients, whichever occupational group they are representing. This has been particularly challenging for staff, all of whom have risen well to the task.

Patient groups

The Ealing ICS "is aimed at any adult where there is deterioration in physical health, function and/or social circumstances which puts them at risk of admission or re-admission to hospital, but where there is actually no over-riding medical reason for admission. This would include those people seen to be at risk because their primary carer is ill but likely to be able to resume their caring role within a short period of time".[13] Criteria for referral are: residency in Ealing Borough; medical stability (though they may have a minor medical problem); a social or functional need which is likely to precipitate hospital admission; and an expectation of return to their previous level of independence within 4-6 weeks.

Evaluation

Figures collected since the introduction of the Intermediate Care scheme indicate that it has had a significant impact on patient services in Ealing.

Figure 2 *(page 14)* shows the number of patients seen by the core assessment team in A&E or in the community between July and December of 1998, alongside those who received a major package of care. The latter can be taken as the number of admissions which have been prevented.

Twenty-one respite beds were supported financially between July and October 1998 with an estimated save of 882 bed days, on the premise that these patients would have needed a six week stay in hospital.

---

[13] Intermediate Care Newsheet. Issue 1, September/October 1998

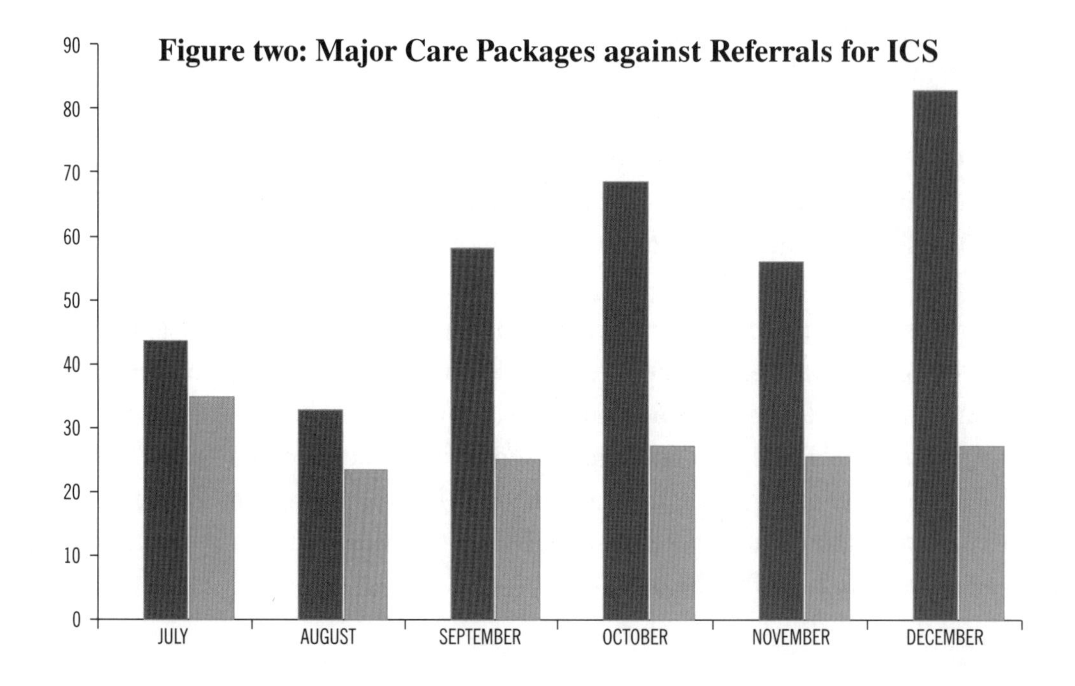

In addition, in any one week there has been an average of 9.7 people being supported by the Stepdown scheme, and between eight and 11 people as part of the post discharge rehabilitation scheme each month.

An estimate of the overall number of bed days which have been saved for the acute Trust has been made between July and December of 1998 using the figures given above. These suggest that Ealing would have needed a further 48 beds in order to accommodate the needs of the local population if the Intermediate Care programme had not been in place. In addition, rehabilitation of patients while under the care of ICS has improved their function and therefore reduced their on-going level of dependence. This has financial savings for social services; early estimates suggest £480,000 pa.

Why has it worked?

From the outset, time and effort has been spent in ensuring that key players are 'on board'. There is a multi professional, Ealing Whole Systems steering group with additional representation from the adjoining boroughs of Hammersmith and Hounslow. The clinical director sits on the hospital executive board and on a social service management board, and there is joint accountability to both organisations. There is also joint investment.

Collaboration, commitment, willingness to take risks and opportunistic funding are all seen to have contributed to the success of the scheme. Lack of planning time, tribalism, divided loyalties and uncertainty have been threatening. The major issue has, since the outset, been handling the interface.

Funding

In the early days funding came from a number of different sources including Tomlinson and Challenge funds, alongside mainstream contributions from both health and social services. The team have also been successful in securing 1997/8 winter pressure money, which, while presenting a considerable challenge in terms of the speed with which the developments were launched, also allowed for further flexible developments.

A further business case has been submitted to the major stakeholders, based on the evidence to date, to continue the service as an independent directorate and to secure the majority of funding from mainstream. In the future, active involvement will be sought from PCGs both for funding and for the strategic development of the service.

Contact details

Dr Janet Ballard
Clinical Director
Intermediate Care Service
Ealing Hospital NHS Trust
Southall, Middx UB1 3HW
Tel: 0181 967 5777

Mr Steve Barnes
Service Manager
Intermediate Care Service
Ealing Hospital NHS Trust
Southall, Middx UB1 3HW
Tel: 0181 967 5663

Manchester – Intermediate care services

Purpose of the service

The South Manchester Intermediate Care service was developed in the spring of 1997 with the primary purpose of facilitating early discharge from hospital. Based on the premise that there was a group of patients who would be as well or better served if their discharge could be accelerated, a pilot scheme was introduced to assess the viability and efficacy of this type of care. This Intermediate Care service is now being rolled out throughout Manchester alongside a range of other options.

Context

Manchester Health Authority was successful in bidding for Challenge Fund money in January of 1997 with a specific remit to explore admission prevention. In order to achieve this objective they brought together a group of GPs who were known to be innovative in their approaches to care. Consensus was reached within the group that early efforts would be concentrated on accelerating discharge since the client group who would benefit by the new service would already have been through the process of hospital assessment, would have a clear medical diagnosis and be known as (relatively) medically stable. As a starting point this group was seen as 'safer' to manage in the community than those whose admission might be prevented, but it would still achieve the objective of taking some pressure off acute beds.

A pilot site in South Manchester was identified to take this work forward, chosen in relation to a series of contextual issues including:

- the recent development of an out-of-hours 'co operative' by a local group of GPs
- interest by the Acute Trust in participating. The medical director had a background in general practice and was sensitive to the potential for such a scheme. The Trust also had major financial pressures and the Health Authority was keen to support any initiative which would lighten this burden
- the Community Trust had already piloted small admission prevention schemes and demonstrated a keen interest in further developments.

Concurrently the Health Authority had commissioned an audit of emergency admissions for the winter of 1996/7[14]. Results indicated a city wide problem of admissions which could potentially have been avoided by a greater capacity within community services to sustain care at home. It was estimated that 8% of medical admissions could have been handled differently if alternative services had been available and that, for 60% of inpatients, there was at least a one-day delay in

---

[14] HaCCRU (1997) *Manchester Emergency Medical Admissions Audit* The Health and Community Care Research Unit, Manchester

discharge. This report has been influential in later developments as it provides clear evidence of local need.

Thus it was the amalgamation of a number of different driving forces, arising out of a range of different contextual issues specific to the locality, which set the scheme on its way.

Getting going

A stakeholder meeting of local GPs, and locality, acute trust and health authority managers was held to explore a potential model for transfer of care which would be adopted for the project. The initial approach, driven by the Health Authority, made use of a team of general practitioners employed as Intermediate Care Physicians working in an outreach capacity from the acute trust. The Health Authority had some initial concern about the quality of care delivered by the local Deputising Service who provided overnight care between 11pm and 7am and did not want to overload this service further. However the General Practitioners were clear that these concerns were unfounded and that they would prefer to manage their own patients' care rather than introduce another 'layer' into the system. Hence it was agreed that they would accept responsibility for medical management of care once patients were transferred back to the community. Their concern about the employment of physicians specifically for the project also, to some extent, acted as a driver for the local GPs in taking on board the new service themselves.

An alternative model, with GP participation, was developed but, since there was high pressure to establish a service very quickly because of the imperative to spend Challenge Fund money by the end of the financial year, GPs were asked to 'sign up' within the week. The speed with which the scheme was being driven again created concern, this time with the LMC but this was resolved with the move to a clinician led scheme introduced in a more manageable time scale. It was agreed that the management protocol which the GPs were to follow was over and above the normal General Medical Services provision. A small additional management fee was agreed to be paid from the Challenge fund budget in recognition of the additional commitment. The project was then relaunched with the local Acute and Community Trusts, alongside 16 (that is 55%) of the local GP practices, who signed up to the scheme. Social services support was initially secured through subcontracting to an independent agency.

Staffing and support

Initially an additional nurse assessor was employed to work alongside the discharge liaison nurses to identify patients in acute care who might be suitable to enter the scheme. If discharge home was not possible, arrangements were made to spot purchase nursing home beds as a step down facility. However this option is no longer used as it was found to be both costly and clinically inappropriate since it necessitated an additional change in venue for the patients to deal with.

Over time this staffing profile shifted as the multiple purpose of some of the roles led to confusion around the manner in which the admission protocols were used. After a two month period the liaison team returned to their original role and an additional Intermediate Care assessor was employed to ensure continuity of service, particularly for sickness and annual leave cover.

Home care was provided by local district nursing services, who, despite initial concerns about workload, had sufficient back up systems provided through bank and agency support, to manage the change. Links between the acute and community teams provided any additional skills training for the nurses. Additional therapy support (0.5 of an occupational therapist and a physiotherapist) were involved from the outset. In addition social care was available, initially through an independent agency.

Medical cover is supplied by the patients own GPs. All patients are visited within one working day of discharge. On average each patient is seen twice. The number of emergency calls over the first year has been minimal.

Patient groups and numbers

The Intermediate Care team estimated that they could deal with around 14 patients a week, a figure based as much on the financial constraints of the project and a feel for the size of the population as more formal data. The service is now working to capacity. The increasing numbers can partly be attributed to a growing awareness of the scheme as well as the increased confidence of those concerned and hence a willingness to take people into Intermediate Care with greater clinical needs.

Early patients were most frequently referred from the orthopaedic unit while the medical unit, despite acute pressure on beds, has been slower to refer. The patients who have presented the greatest challenge have been those referred from the vascular surgery unit which can readily be explained by the greater degree of underlying pathology which initially led them to need surgical intervention. It is worth noting that since the inception of the scheme there have only been 4 night calls and only 24, from a total of 330 patients, have required readmission.

Admission criteria to the scheme include:

- Manchester resident
- patient consent
- GP signed up to the scheme
- likely to be able to return to previous level of independence with up to 14 days of support from nurses and therapists and 28 days of social care

Why has it worked?

The Health Authority has identified a series of reasons which it considers have contributed to the success of this scheme. These include:

- leadership and support of the scheme from its inception onwards
- identification of clinical champions including a local general practitioner and the Health Authority medical director
- commitment of local financial resources
- knowledge of real problems through auditing of local need [15]
- appointment of a dedicated project manager to undertake the managerial leg work
- time to mature without giving up
- promotion of successes locally and nationally

From the General Practitioners' perspective the scheme has gained success because:

- they consider it better for the patients
- clinical management of the patients has not proved either too difficult or too different from previous work
- the small payment gave symbolic recognition to their commitment
- one-to-one liaison between the hospital staff and GPs ensured that they had accurate up to date information
- the option of not accepting an early discharge referral gave them control over the degree of complex clinical need which they felt comfortable to manage

In addition a bi-monthly newsletter, initiated by the lead GP and widely circulated, ensured raised awareness and regular feedback, as well as providing a means of demonstrating a valuing of the positive contribution of the programme.

Evaluation

Audit data has been recorded from the outset of this scheme by the Clinical Audit Departments of the Acute and Community Trusts. Data in relation to costs has been gathered and analysed by Manchester Health Authority and the Trusts. Results to date include:

Number seen	330 over first 18 months, including the small numbers dealt with at the outset of the service
Night visits	4
Readmissions	3-4%
LoS	professionally estimated according to need
Clinical need	no greater than general discharge needs
Patient satisfaction	five case studies have been undertaken, all of which have shown a high level of patient satisfaction

[15] HaCCRU (1997) op cit

What next?

In the spring of 1998 Manchester Health Authority undertook a mapping exercise of local services. This confirmed their view that, while there were a large number of pilot initiatives throughout the city, many of which provided excellent local facilities, there was a lack of cohesiveness and a risk that new developments may overlap or fail to survive as the 'product champions' moved on. The care task force were keen that a whole systems approach would be taken to bring together all the resources available in a co-ordinated manner. Additional 'whole systems' funding[16], targeted at reducing waiting lists, was used to introduce a city wide strategy, known colloquially as 'Jigsaw' and more fully as 'Consolidating Partnerships for Best Practice' (Figure three)

Figure three - Consolidating Partnerships for Best Practice

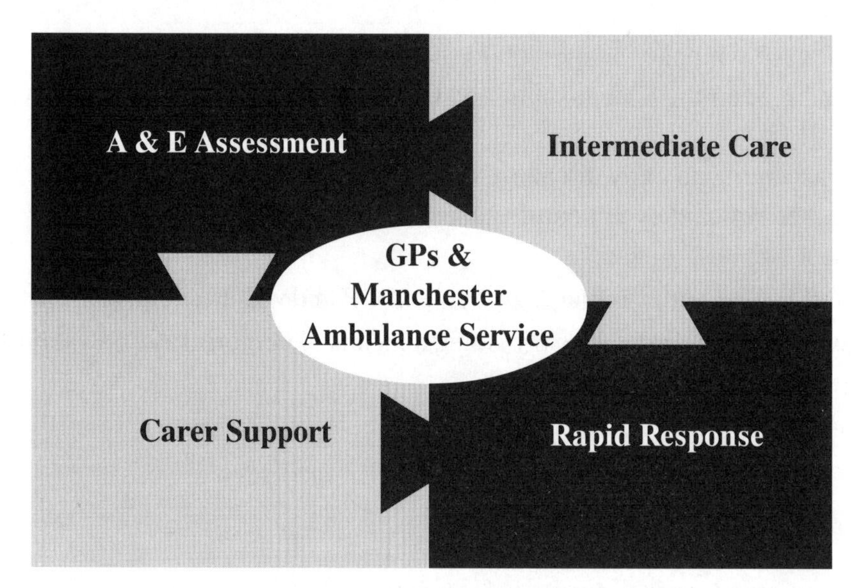

The plan has four key arms:

1. Roll-out of the intermediate care work described above to central and north Manchester
2. Further development of a small rapid response scheme aimed at keeping people who need short term support but not specialist medical intervention, in their own homes. Up to 48 hours of health and social care can be put in place by the rapid response team, to allow time for further services to be activated for up to 14 days. There is a 'mix and match' of provision for social care between social services and the independent sector. An interesting development which has arisen from this scheme has been the need to help social care workers to promote independence rather than offering a specific ongoing service, in line with recommendations of the Modernising Social Services report[17]. This has required that they learn a new way of working. Hence it has been necessary to develop a new training package. Options in the longer term are also being explored to undertake more joint assessments, prepare multi skilled care

---

[16] Whole systems money

[17] Department of Health (1998) *Modernising social services: Promoting independence, Improving protection, Raising standards* London DoH

workers and therapy assistants and review the team skillmix.

3. In the light of the HaCCRU findings a city wide pilot has been introduced in Manchester to divert inappropriate admissions through A and E with the help of a rapid response team. Assessment by the Intermediate Care assessor, in collaboration with the district nursing liaison team, of patients referred from A and E staff will hopefully lead to admission prevention for this group with appropriate home care packages being offered instead.
4. With an eye to the risk of additional pressure on home carers, Cross Roads (a voluntary organisation) is providing additional carer support, through trained care assistants offering respite care in patients' own homes.

These services are co-ordinated through a central control base. They can be accessed through a single phone call. Plans are underway to co-locate the control centre with the social services emergency duty out of hours team.

Funding

These developments have been funded throughout with soft, non-recurring money, initially through Challenge Funds which, with some slippage, will be available until April 2000. Winter pressure money has allowed an increase in the community nursing resource, recognising that additional resources are needed for Intermediate Care to be able to respond to the care shift from acute to primary care. Skill mix is also being reviewed in primary and community care. One option under consideration is to increase the practice nurse role in relation to preventative services for older people. In this way the distribution of work between general practitioners, community nurses and therapists and social services can be adjusted as the demand increases.

There is a view that the success of the schemes has, to some extent, been influenced by the fact that they have not so far encroached on central funding. Thus, to date, there has been no cost loss, which may have necessitated cuts to the traditional services. Whether or not this is sustainable is under question and current discussions with the local Trusts and the Regional office are underway to consider priorities and service contracts.

Contact details

Peter Fink
Director of Intermediate Care
The Maples Medical Centre
2 Scout Drive
Newell Green
Manchester
M23 2SY
Tel: 0161 498 8484

Mandy Wearne
Director of Development
Manchester Health Authority
Gateway House
Piccadilly South
Manchester
M60 7LP
Tel: 0161 237 2090

Department for the Medicine of Ageing at Chelsea & Westminster Hospital Day Medicine Unit

Aims of the Unit

The Chelsea and Westminster Day Medicine Unit is part of the Chelsea and Westminster NHS Trust. It was formally opened in March 1998. The primary purpose of the unit is to offer a service to the local population which can, through timely early intervention, reduce the need for admission; prevent deterioration whenever possible; and, help elderly people especially to maintain maximum independence and quality of life at home. The three key features are:

- a link between primary and secondary care
- general practitioner support and education
- increasing the profile of elderly care

The unit is needs driven and based on a fundamental belief that there must be a shift from the traditional 'prosthetic' approach in service delivery (where problems are merely patched up when they arise) to one which encompasses short and long term action by early intervention and active prevention. In this way care can be pushed 'up stream' with, for example, early attention to prevention of falls and osteoporosis reducing, in the longer term, the number of older people suffering from fractures. Thus the unit focuses on both rapid access for early assessment and support, and longer term preventative strategies. Within this process the critical role of expert early assessment, with appropriate consultant-led diagnosis, supported by a multi-professional perspective, is seen as the bedrock of good practice.

Context

Chelsea and Westminster is set in central London, serving a population of some 160,000 people of whom 4,000 (2.5%) are aged over 80 years (national average (~2 %). Forty per cent of general practices are singled handed and there is very low use of residential beds in the immediate locality. It is estimated that over the next decade the locally served population of those aged over 80 years will increase to 6,000 (3.75%). Thus service providers are presented with a demographic dilemma – those aged over 80 years are already big users of hospital in-patient services – and this is exacerbated by other contextual issues that began in the sixties; such as the change in the abortion law and access to contraception impacting on the size of the potential work force through the nineties and into the millennium.[18]

In 1995 the whole Medicine directorate faced significant difficulties in managing the number of all-

---

[18] Livesley J, Wallace S, Livesley B (1992) *Towards a social policy on ageing: a consultation report.* Kent: The Research for Ageing Trust

age adult patients in their care. These were frequently placed as 'outliers' throughout the hospital, with the familiar knock-on effects for general surgery and orthopaedics. Early steps were taken to break this cycle by fully integrating general and geriatric medicine and creating an admissions ward. Within a year the team were successful not only in reducing the number of outliers (Figure four), but also in decreasing the average length of stay, hence increasing productivity (Figure five). Over time the demand for beds was reduced but it was recognised that there would be seasonal variations. A 'summer-winter share' of beds was negotiated with the surgical directorate which has enabled bed numbers, and hence staffing, to be maintained throughout thc ycar but with an appropriate variation in activity.

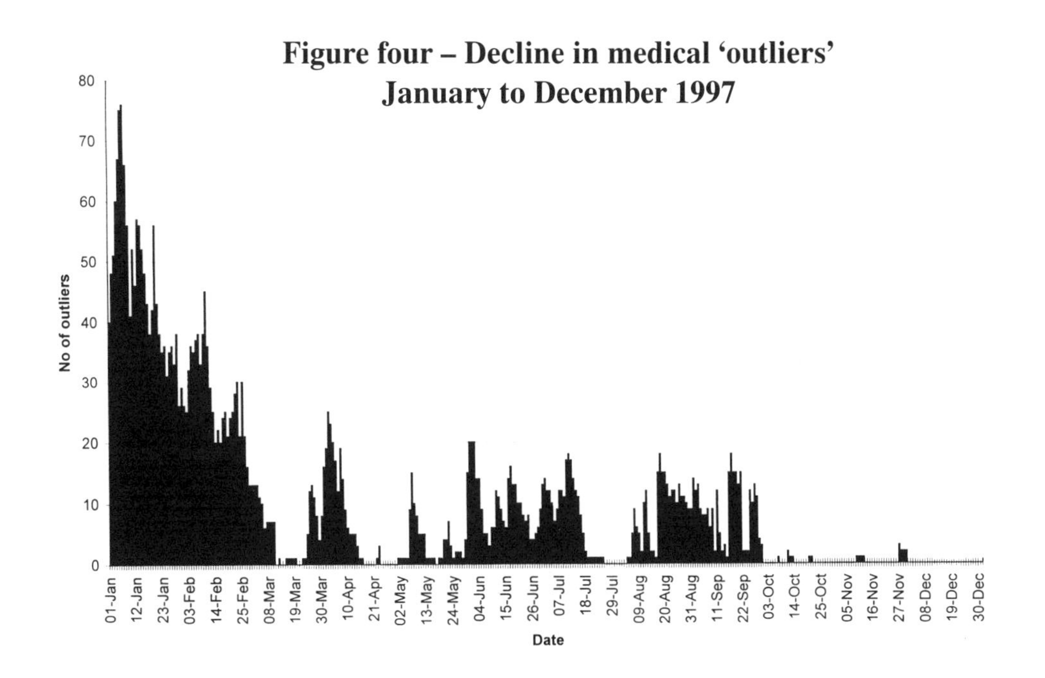

Figure four – Decline in medical 'outliers' January to December 1997

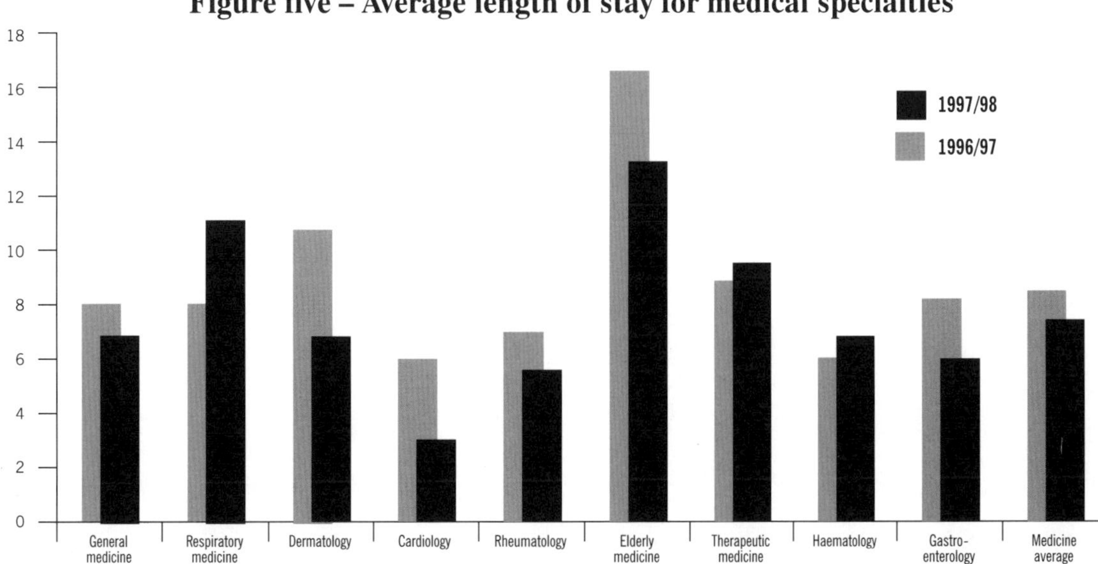

Figure five – Average length of stay for medical specialties

However, with an activity forecast of increasing demand over the next decade the team recognised pragmatically, economically, and philosophically, that further action would be needed. Since the interface between acute and primary care was a critical factor in this situation a questionnaire was distributed to local general practitioners to ascertain what type of services would be most valuable to them. There was a premise that if admission could be prevented and people could go home in a better position to manage their own lives then the long term demand on beds could be reduced further. The high response rate to the questionnaire (60%) demonstrated in itself the relevance of taking a new look at services and indicated priorities in:

- consultant access
- speed of access and telephone referrals
- hassle free hospital admissions
- 'complete services' (health and social care)
- specialist services
- continuing community care for frail elderly people

In order to meet these challenges it was agreed that a new range of services would be introduced primarily providing day (or ambulatory) care and, as far as possible, they would be combined into a one-stop-service for the convenience of patients attending.

The Day Medicine Unit

Client group

General practitioners, community nurses, and accident & emergency staff can make direct referrals to the unit for rapid assessment or access to one of the unit's specialist services (see below). While the majority of clients are in an older age group of 70 years and upwards, there is an increasing number of referrals for younger people. This is in line with the focus of the unit on the process of ageing rather than the concept of old age. Figure six gives an indication of the increase in the number of day-care contacts over the past three years.

Figure six – The increase in the number of day-care contacts over the past three years

1996/7	468 day patients
1997/8	876 day patients
1998/9	1008 day patients

Access to the services is directed through the medical team driven by the strong commitment to expert early assessment by a medical consultant. The rationale behind this decision is based on a belief that expert medical assessment is critical for effective clinical diagnosis to be made, in order to ensure that the right programme of care is offered. There is also a concern that para-clinical team members would not have the broad diagnostic skills of medicine, which may not only jeopardise patient care but also place the practitioners at risk medico-legally, if they see patients with undifferentiated diagnoses.

Range of services

Services have been developed in line with the requests from general practitioners alongside the expert knowledge of the acute care team. These services are steadily expanding but currently encompass:

Rapid response service – a consultant assessment can be obtained within three working days which may divert emergency admissions while assuring that patients have access to specialist expertise.

Prevention programmes/clinics (e.g. Falls, TIAs) – these programmes also work on the premise that, wherever possible, prevention is a better strategy to follow. The programmes focus on preventing or limiting potential problems. Direct referrals from the accident and emergency department occur commonly, particularly to the Falls clinic.

Specialist clinics for chronic disease management (e.g. heart failure, stroke, Alzheimer's disease, Parkinson's disease) – this service offers help and advice on clinical management as well as the social challenges which arise for these patients but are often put to one side as being 'too hard to handle'.

Help line facilities – these services are offered to patients, general practitioners, and carers in response to market research. They work on the premise that a timely word of advice can divert a problem or expedite action. Replies are sent to general practitioners' surgeries by same-day telephone or fax or, in other cases, by letter the following day.

Multidisciplinary 'bridging team' – this on-site team provides a 24 hour emergency service throughout each week (supported by the Riverside Night Nursing service between 8pm to 8am) for patients at risk of hospital admission due to functional deterioration. Patients referred to this service must require only simple care assistance (e.g. basic hygiene needs, meal provision, removal of sutures and dressings). Up to five days of such care in the community can be provided to resettle patients after discharge from hospital, and allow time for a more formal community package to be established with other services including physiotherapy and occupational therapy. The 'bridging team' has created an essential network relationship with community and social care services including those outside the borough.

Day medical care provision – this service resembles day surgery care in that treatments which have previously only been offered as part of inpatient care can now be offered through ambulatory day care facilities. Examples include administration of chemotherapy and blood transfusions.

Flexible clinics – some clinics are established according to seasonal need such as a 'Winter Chest Clinic' for patients predisposed to exacerbations of bronchitis, that would otherwise precipitate hospital admission. This provision will increasingly encompass palliative care for non-cancerous conditions including pre-terminal heart and respiratory failure.

A knock-on effect of the introduction of these clinics has been an opportunity for general practitioners to update their knowledge of some specialist aspects of practice, by receiving prompt information about their patients. In consequence, and over time, it has been found that patient need can be handled with greater confidence in the community (viz. the management of chronic heart failure) giving the Day Medicine Unit the capacity to expand into other areas of care.

The shape of the team

Since its inception the Medicine of Ageing department has acknowledged that teamwork (encompassing both clinical, para-clinical, and managerial staff) is an essential component of modern medicine. Over time the team has been shaped and developed by the lead consultant to meet the changing needs of the patients. It now consists of five other consultant physicians, senior nurses, physio- and occupational-therapists, the manager of the medicine directorate and her deputy, and a finance officer. Each of the physicians shares in the hospital's acute-medical on-take and also the Day Medicine unit's rapid response service. In addition, one of the physicians is leading liaison with the community interface, continuing care, and non-stroke neurology; another physician leads liaison for the medical-orthopaedic-A&E service and the falls and heart failure clinics; one is involved in stroke management; one leads the medical input into the surgical services and the spina bifida clinic; and the newest physician (who is not on acute-take) is developing palliative care for patients with non-cancerous conditions.

There is a marked emphasis on staff development with team members from all disciplines taking an active part in both internal learning opportunities and external programmes. There is a ten-year track record of academic achievement, to masters and doctorate levels, for paramedical and junior medical staff and the team have published widely. Special part-time research posts were introduced historically to raise standards in the paramedical fields and a nursing development unit was established. The culture is one of learning and research which has been developed over time.

The work of the unit is also reflected in the undergraduate medical curriculum where a greater emphasis on the management of ageing and care of older people was introduced some time ago.

Funding

Much of the initial funding for this unit came from soft, non-recurring money, through initiatives such as LIZ, Tomlinson and, more recently, the Winter Beds fund. The community liaison and medical-orthopaedic services were developed as a part of the pre-formed business plans. The NHS

Health Trust was persuaded to create short-term locum-consultant posts to undertake clinical audit programmes in their respective areas. These clearly demonstrated the success of these initiatives. For example, the medical-orthopaedic-A&E service saved the Trust some £350,000 in its first year as the average duration of stay of elderly orthopaedic patients was reduced by over 25%, from 23 to 17 days. This enabled better use of much needed clinical facilities.

Evaluation

An ongoing evaluation of the Day Medicine unit forms part of the wider research programme of the team and it is already possible to see changes in activity, length of stay, and patterns of referral from general practitioners. There is also an indication that admissions are being diverted and readmissions reduced. For example, data available from the Falls clinic shows that for every five new patients seen one admission is prevented. This reduction of 24 admissions over a one year period corresponds to 480 bed-days saved.

However the team are clear that it will take a further two/three years before the impact of the Day Medicine unit will be fully realised and even then the context will be continuing to change. Hence the data they have been able to gather to date can only begin to throw light on the clinical and economic efficacy of the unit. It does, however, show promising trends and within the clinical effectiveness arena the developments are based on 'best evidence available'.

The process of implementation

This has taken time – the service was first envisaged more than five years ago. First, potential consultant physicians were specially recruited and supported in locum-posts working towards a pre-formed business plan. Then the needs of the purchasers (mainly local general practitioners) were identified and services were shaped to ensure and monitor patient satisfaction. Having defined the aims of the service, teams were developed to respond to the needs of patients. The resulting opportunities allowed team members to achieve personal satisfaction and career development in their roles. This encouraged the development of an important morale factor. Each aspect of the developing service came under a physician leader – each of whom had been trained within the department and developed the ability 'to learn what needs to be done by doing and leading what needs to be learned'. These leaders have acquired a helicopter view of what is being achieved within their part of the service. This has been aided by clinical audit and the need to give regular presentations to others (both at under- and post-graduate levels at lectures, seminars, etc.) on behalf of the department as a whole.

Finally, there is no concern expressed about ownership when aspects of the department's service grow sufficiently to become autonomous. It is already apparent that some activities within the department are going to become subspecialties in their own right because of the core knowledge they are acquiring. These may follow the example of the patients' discharge-facilitation team. This was initially soft-money funded by the department but has now extended to serve the whole hospital.

The future

The day medicine unit is continuously changing and developing in response to both clinical and contextual demands. The demand on some services is already reducing as a higher level of current knowledge and hence safe care, has been passed on to colleagues working in the community. In this way capacity can be created within the unit to further develop the range of services offered.

The combination of intermediate and ambulatory care services is already expanding and reaching a wider proportion of the population as this type of service is being taken up by other disciplines, notably chemotherapy and clinical haematology.

Contact details

Professor Brian Livesley
The University of London's Professor in the Care of the Elderly
Imperial College School of Medicine
Chelsea & Westminster Hospital
369 Fulham Road
London SW10 9NH
Tel: 0181 746 8063
Fax: 0181 746 8183

Cass Ward – Homerton Hospital

Nurse-led In-patient beds

Background and purpose

Cass ward is a nurse-led in-patient service situated in an acute district general hospital in the East End of Inner London. It is a 19 bedded unit which focuses on offering care to patients whose medical condition has stabilised but who have the potential to improve the quality of their lives and degree of independence through the intensive support of nurses, while retaining the same amount of access to therapy services as elsewhere in the hospital.

Context

The decision to introduce a nurse-led unit was taken in 1995, at a time when there was high pressure on acute beds; in the winter months patients were having to remain on trolleys over night in the Accident and Emergency Department (with one incident recorded of 25 patients on trolleys in a single night); and emergency admissions were on the increase. It was acknowledged that there was a need for at least 20 extra beds which the Health Authority agreed to fund.

The natural inclination at that time was to introduce a new medical ward. However consideration was given to the findings of the 1992 Audit Commission report[19] which suggested that around 48% of people occupying medical beds at that time did not require the full range of services of an acute unit. This was coupled with the fact that the hospital already had a track record of innovations in nursing with well developed nurse practitioner roles and nurse-led services. A case was made that an alternative solution would be the introduction of a nurse-led ward, replicating the Dulwich model[20].

An audit of the hospital in-patient population indicted that there were between 20 and 30 patients at any one time who would meet the criteria for the unit (see below) and an initial costing exercise appeared favourable. Difficulty was also being experienced at that time in maintaining junior medical staff cover as the recommendations of New Deal[21] were implemented. These factors, alongside the active support of the Chief Executive for innovations of this nature, led to a decision that a nurse-led unit would be the optimum solution. A proposal was presented to the Health Authority, confirming that there was an appropriate patient group, that the model should be cost efficient and that it could potentially lead to better clinical outcomes. The proposal was approved and plans made to proceed.

---

[19] Audit Commission (1992) *Lying in Wait: The Use of Medical Beds in Acute Hospitals* London HMSO

[20] Evans A, Griffiths P (1994) *The Development of a Nursing-led In-patient Service* London King's Fund

[21] Department of Health (1991) *Hours of work for doctors in training: the new deal* London DoH (EL(91)82)

Getting going

At the outset a project nurse was employed with sole responsibility to develop the unit. In addition the views and comments of all the potential stakeholders were sought. A major communication strategy was developed across the Trust to ensure that colleagues were aware of the existence of the unit and its prime purpose of reducing pressure on acute beds, while providing a needs specific service for a well defined group of patients. An operational policy was drawn up encompassing:

Referral processes – a senior medical colleague may refer a patient who will then be assessed by a member of the Cass nursing team within the following 24 hours. Specific admission criteria have been developed against which the assessment is made.

Admission criteria include:

- medically stable for at least 24 hours
- no significant changes in medical management anticipated
- patient could potentially benefit from active nursing intervention in one or more of the following – education/psychological care/re-mobilisation/symptom control/nutrition/feeding/ wound care/ nurturing
- routine investigations (bloods and ECG) are available and, where any abnormalities are present, a course of action agreed
- discharge destination has been identified
- a stay of more than 4 further days is envisaged
- a medical opinion on any unexplained anaemia has been obtained
- the patient is over 16 and has given verbal consent for transfer

The purpose behind this process is to ensure that the patients who are referred to the unit have already been subject to expert medical assessment, are not likely to need further medical intervention as an in-patient, but are likely to benefit from the specific services of the team. The criteria also ensure exclusion of patients who would not benefit by transfer. Once transferred to Cass the patient is 'discharged' from the care of the consultant and a new episode of care is commenced.

Initially the unit was sited in a ward that had become available following the relocation of another unit to a new building. It has since been re-housed to a quieter 19 bedded site within the hospital with more friendly surroundings, and a setting which is more conducive to the philosophy of care.

Staffing profile and development

Staff were recruited specifically to work on Cass. Indeed one of the rationale for the development of this service was to aid nurse recruitment which was historically difficult in this location. The principle was to develop a 'Magnet Hospital'[22] culture of motivation and excellence which is supported further by the hospital's commitment to staff development. Appointments were made through both internal promotion and external advertising but the process took longer than had originally been anticipated and had to go to several rounds. Staffing on Cass is now stable but remains an area which requires continuous effort to attract appropriately qualified and skilled nursing staff.

The team is made up of:

1 (clinical) leader	'H' grade
1 ward facilitator	'G' grade
3 primary nurses	'F' grade
3 associate nurses	'E' grade
6 associate nurses	'D' grade
1 healthcare support worker	'A' grade

Service contracts have been agreed with occupational therapy for one WTE, alongside support from the senior OT; 0.2 WTE physiotherapist and helper; and one social worker dedicated to the unit. Standard speech therapy support is also available.

Medical cover is provided by a general practitioner who gives eight hours service each week. Initially the GP did a 'round' of all the patients receiving nurse-led care on each visit but, as confidence and competence have increased, this practice has shifted and the GP only sees those patients referred by the nurse. The nurses can initiate investigations, including routine blood tests and urine and sputum analysis, prior to the GP visit, in order to ensure that there is no delay in treatment being instigated. Emergency cover is available through the hospital on call system.

As the unit opened the primary nurses undertook a module in patient assessment run at King's College University over a three month period (a day a week). However the majority of additional skills, such as chest percussion, were acquired on site with the help of medical colleagues and the units medical officer. Some 'extended role' skills, such as cannulation and certification of expected death, where taught by the night nurse practitioners.

An in-house health care assistant programme which leads to awarding of NVQ level two and three certificates is also available.

Patients

Currently bed occupancy runs at 98% on Cass and 60% of patients receive the nurse led service. Thus 11 of the beds are occupied by patients with nurse-led needs, the remainder being used for patients with medical needs. This relatively small number does not reflect the potential population identified in the original audit and may be a reflection of the increase in rehabilitation activity in

---

[22] Buchan J (1997) 'Magnet hospitals: what's the attraction? *Nursing Standard* 12 (7) 22-25

the elderly care unit. It has led the unit to reconsidering and widening the admission criteria to encompass those patients with needs which are sensitive to skilled nursing including:

- patients with complex discharge problems
- facilitated discharge following orthopaedic medical treatment
- palliative care
- some respite care

The diagnostic category of the current patient group is wide ranging encompassing patients with, among others, muscula-skeletal, cardiac, gastro-intestinal, gentio-urinary and respiratory problems[23]. A break down of the nursing needs of the patients who have been cared for in the unit is given in Figure seven.

Figure seven - Nursing needs/reason for referral of patients cared for on Cass ward

Category of Nursing Need	Number treated on Cass
Wound care	11 (13%)
Symptom control	7 (8%)
Remoblisation	84 (98%)
Psychological	11 (13%)
Nutrition/feeding	11 (13%)
Nurturing	23 (27%)
Education	9 (10%)
N=86	
NB Most patients had more than one nursing need	

The majority of patients (79% over a period of 8 months – N=70) were originally admitted to hospital from either their own, or warden controlled homes. No transfers were accepted of patients who had been admitted from nursing homes.

Evaluation

Funds were sought at the outset of this project from the North Thames Research and Development programme to undertake formal evaluation. A randomised controlled trial,

[23] for further breakdown see *Substitution of 'Nursing-led In-patient Units' (NLIUs) for Acute Services* Homerton Hospital NHS Trust London, Division of Nursing and Midwifery, King's College London and York Centre for Health Economics University of York.

replicating the methodology developed to evaluate the Dulwich unit [24] was employed, focusing on clinical and economic outcomes. Patient satisfaction, multi- professional team work and processes of care were also explored. The full report is available elsewhere[25] but some key findings and their impact are included here.

A total of 175 patients entered the study, 89 of whom formed the treatment group while 86 were in the control group. The variable used was transfer to the nurse-led unit. No significant differences were found in the two groups against age, sex, functional independence, ethnicity, medical diagnosis or nursing need. Of the factors studied no significant difference was found in discharge destination, complications (such as chest or urinary infections), rates of readmission or mortality. The treatment group showed a trend to greater improvement in all psychometric measures employed including Bartel index, GHQ12 and NHPD. However, length of stay was longer, leading to a higher overall cost per hospital stay although costs per day were lower.

Since the results for length of stay were made available the nurse-led unit has taken steps to reverse this trend. At the time of the study they did not have access to the hospital discharge team's services so were potentially under served in this support service. They have now increased their formal links with the social worker to precipitate appropriate packages of home care more speedily. Weekly discharge forums, alongside clinical supervision, have been introduced for each primary nurse to help them gain skills and confidence in discharge planning. Case loads are monitored every 15 days. Since these steps have been taken the average stay in the unit has been reduced to 22 days on an annual calculation and 10 days over the last recorded month. The 22 day figure is calculated formally through the hospital's information department. The 10 day figure is purely for one month and has been calculated by the primary nurses and is not, at the time of reporting, cumulative.

In relation to patient satisfaction treatment group patients and their families were more satisfied on all factors studied but none of these findings was significant.

The staffing profile on the unit showed a high proportion of senior nursing staff but an overall lower proportion of qualified staff. The overall ratio of nurses to patients was lower than elsewhere in the hospital (0.44 nurses/ patient – mean 0.63). Less input from professions allied to medicine was evident in the treatment group which may have contributed to the greater length of stay.

Cost per day was lower in the nurse-led unit than elsewhere but overall costs were significantly higher owing to the greater length of stay. Intervention costs were neutral, while post discharge costs were lower in the treatment group. Correction in the length of stay on the nurse-led unit will have had a self-evident impact on current costs.

---

[24] Griffiths P, Evans A (1995) Evaluating a nursing-led in-patient service: an interim report London King's Fund

[25] *Substitution of 'Nursing-led In-patient Units' (NLIUs) for Acute Services* (1998) op cit

Funding

At the time that the unit was established it was agreed that the cost would be no greater than a comparable medical ward, estimated at £965,121 per annum. In reality the unit costs per annum are around £837,260 (for staff and non staff costs), showing a difference of £127,861. Evaluation costs were found elsewhere (see above) and staff development was subsumed within the hospital framework.

The Future

Since the initial concern about the costing data Cass has dramatically reduced its average length of stay for patients and has demonstrated that it is a viable complimentary service for a designated group of patients. It has been agreed that the unit will continue to run for the foreseeable future, aiming to increase the number of beds occupied by patients receiving nurse-led care and continuing to address the overall length of stay. Both these achievements are already well on the way to being achieved.

In addition it is recognised that some of the practices which have been developed on Cass, such as self medication programmes for the patients, are being taken up elsewhere in the hospital and it is hoped that the unit will continue to act as a pilot site for the development of other practices such as the clinical decision making process and the development of evidence based standards.

The unit is already taking patients with a slightly greater degree of need, reflecting the increased confidence of the nursing team. Other intermediate initiatives are also being developed in the Trust, including a newly introduced children's service targeted at keeping children at home whenever possible (see directory entry p 103).

Contact details

Therese Davis
Director of Nursing and Quality

Homerton Hospital NHS Trust
Homerton Row
London E9 6SR
Tel: 0181 510 7321

Heather Ferguson
Senior Nurse for the Directorate of Medicine and Out Patients
Homerton Hospital NHS Trust
Homerton Row
London E9 6SR
Tel: 0181 510 7840

Sir Alfred Jones Memorial Hospital
North Mersey Community NHS Trust

Background and purpose of the service

Sir Alfred Jones Memorial Hospital, which was originally built as a fever hospital in 1869, is sited in Garston on the outskirts of Liverpool. It was endowed by Sir Alfred Jones, a shipping magnet, in 1913. There are two Nightingale design wards, as well as one double and three single rooms, offering 28 beds in all. The atmosphere is welcoming, albeit in accommodation which has had limited alteration to the main structure since it was first built. The main purpose of the service, which is led by nurse practitioners, is to offer nurse-led inpatient care. Patients are accepted from both the acute Trust and the community against well defined but flexible admission criteria (see below). As the team say, if they think they can make a difference to quality of life for any patient 'in transition' then they will accept him or her. In addition the unit offers a Primary Care Treatment Centre to complement the work of the GPs which is also led by nurse practitioners. A range of minor injuries is treated against well developed protocols with an aim of providing a rapid local service while diverting some pressure from the acute Accident and Emergency department.

Context

Liverpool has a culture of using the hospital as a primary source of treatment, an approach which is exacerbated by the large number of singled handed GP practices in the vicinity. At a time when there was extreme pressure on acute care beds in Liverpool all services were subject to review, including that offered at the Sir Alfred Jones Memorial Hospital. The unit, which was, and still is, held in high regard by the local population, was used exclusively by GPs, mainly for social respite. Bed occupancy was low, around 60%, leaving room for development.

At the same time readmission of discharged patients to the acute service was high and a hospital at home scheme which it had been hoped would relieve some pressure on acute beds had not proved successful. There was general agreement from both the Health Authority and the Community Trust that it was time for change.

The Sir Alfred Jones Memorial Hospital development was part of a wider initiative supported by the Health Authority, who were seeking a package of schemes which would help to bridge between acute and primary care. The impact of the Continuing Care Guidance HSG (95)8 was also an important factor in determining that the hospital should be developed to meet health rather than social care needs. In addition to the community hospital there is a home rehabilitation service, ACTRITE (Acute Chest Triage Rapid Intervention Team), to provide alternative treatment for people with an exacerbation of a chronic chest problem and a range of other admission prevention schemes (see below).

Getting going

A 'stakeholder group' was convened with membership from the local GPs, the CHC, carers, patients, and social services as well as the HA and the Trust, to review options. It was agreed that a service would be established with the following key objectives:

- facilitation of early discharge from acute care
- to maximise support to primary care through integrated rehabilitation
- joint case management (from health and social services)
- GP access to beds to prevent acute admission

There was some pressure to establish a service within a three month time scale but the community Trust negotiated for a much longer run-in time to allow the process of change to be managed well. It was anticipated that there would be a small proportion of people who would find the changes difficult or even unacceptable, requiring some staff redeployment. In addition there were sharp learning curves for all concerned including:

- GPs – who would be using the unit for health rather than social respite
- the acute Trust - in recognising appropriate referrals
- social services - who have since picked up the respite care previously offered in the unit
- the nurses and therapists who had to learn new skills and new ways of working

In addition public meetings were held to ensure that the views of the local community were heard and reassurance was given over specific aspects of concern such as the fear of loss of social respite.

After negotiation it was agreed that the full impact of the unit would not be apparent for up to two years as the transition to a new type of service would take time to become fully operational. This time scale has given the team time to develop both professionally and operationally without unrealistic expectations.

Staffing profile and development

The unit is managed by an H grade nurse, supported by a G grade practice development nurse. In addition there are:

6 Nurse practitioners	(F grade)
7 Care practitioners	(E grade)
11 Support workers	(B grade)

1 WTE Occupational therapist
1 WTE Physiotherapist

0.4 WTE Medical officer
1 WTE Administrator

The initial recruitment process, which was jointly agreed with the Royal College of Nursing and Unison, spanned a two day period with competency assessment at its core, as the quality of the team was essential to the success of the proposed new service. Trade union involvement throughout ensured that there were no staff disputes to handle.

There is no on-site medical cover but the rich skill mix allows for expert nursing cover over the 24 hour period. Admissions and discharges, including length of stay, are managed by the nurse practitioners who have negotiated agreement to refer directly back to the acute Trust, by-passing Accident and Emergency, should the need arise. The data show these referrals to be around 11% of the total number receiving care in the unit.

Medical cover is provided by a local GP with dedicated time for the unit. He has been instrumental in helping the nurse practitioners to recognise their own skills, as well as developing new ones, and to extend their willingness and ability to take responsibility for their own actions. Over time they have felt able to extend the range of decision making which they make independently, as evidenced by the changes in records of the messages left for medical colleague's advice since the unit opened.

An 'in house' needs driven development programme, managed by the occupational therapist, is offered to the support workers (previously nursing assistants) who have developed a generic range of nursing and therapy support skills. Arrangements are also in place for them to achieve NVQs at levels two and three. Thus while the OT and physiotherapist are managed by the senior nurse there are times when they, in turn, manage the nursing support workers. This flexible cross boundary working typifies the way in which the team work together. It has, however, caused some concern with professional colleagues outside the unit, raising interesting questions about the manner in which cross boundary work can be managed on a wider front and the differences in view which arise from an operational and a professional stance.

There is also an 'in house' development programme for E grade Care Practitioners to help them to develop into the Nurse Practitioner role. Discussions are currently underway to gain recognition of this training. In addition, the acute Trust have asked the team to undertake some training with their staff on management of discharge.

There is no recruitment problem in the unit despite major difficulties elsewhere in the locality. Local knowledge that the jobs offer a rewarding and interesting role has ensured that there are multiple applications for any vacancy which does occur although turnover of staff is low. Comments from the staff suggest that there is a demanding but fulfilling role for the nurses and therapists who now find "..life more interesting". For support workers they not only offer a career progression but also a fulfilling holistic role. As one said "We are part of one big family."

Patients

Patients are accepted from the acute Trust or the community in a ratio of about 65 :35. Following referral same day assessment is made by one of the nurse practitioners for suitability and where possible there is immediate transfer. The majority of referrals for April to December 1998 from the acute Trust were as follows:

Medical	28%
Surgical	24%
Orthopaedic	10%

In the early days there was some resistance to admissions being accepted or rejected by nurse practitioners, a difficulty which was overcome by preparation of written admission criteria which were widely circulated. They include:

- age 16 or over
- deemed medically stable for 48 hours minimum
- no significant medical change anticipated
- an anticipated discharge date
- an anticipated discharge destination

Patients are given detailed information about the unit in order to make an informed choice about whether or not they wish to be transferred. They are also screened for M.R.S.A. where appropriate.

The team stress, however, that they must be flexible about the admissions they accept. They did, for example, accept patients who still needed social respite care in the early days in order to help set up more appropriate packages. The main type of patients who have benefited from care in the unit are those who need help with problems such as complex wound healing, rehabilitation following minor stokes, recovery from acute illnesses and help in a safe transition home with confidence. Some palliative and terminal care is also offered, especially when it is the wish of a patient to return to the unit when he or she is dying.

Evaluation

Numerical data is available from the time at which the unit was opened, covering a range of issues including:

Bed occupancy 1997	–	range 40-80% over 12 months
Bed occupancy 1998	–	range 61-96% over 12 months

Bed days saved for acute units April-Dec 1998	–	total 6138 over 9 months
Number of re-admissions	–	42 from 305 over 9 months

Initially there was pressure to undertake a controlled trial to assess the efficacy of the unit and outcomes for the patients. However it was apparent that this methodology would not be appropriate at a time when the unit was developing so rapidly and change was inherent in both the acute Trust and the community hospital. A revised study design, including minimum data sets matched to admission criteria, independence scores, social networks, mini mental state examinations and re-admissions are being collected alongside interview data with staff and patients. Results should be available in the summer.

Funding

The Sir Alfred Jones Memorial Hospital was developed as a cost neutral initiative with no additional money being placed in the unit. Some extra funds have been found for evaluation through the Health Authority. Much of the staff development is covered by the Trust staff training and development department.

The future

The success of the unit has been encouraging locally and there is enthusiasm and commitment to explore other developments. Currently a new Emergency Response Team (ERT) system is being introduced by the community Trust in conjunction with the ambulance service, as a means of offering an alternative to admission for people, seen by the ambulance service, who do not need acute care. The efficacy of a nurse accompanying the ambulance crew is also being assessed currently. The service is supported by health and social services and financed through Challenge Funds. It can provide a package of care for up to 72 hours to allow time to refer into existing services. The most common reason for referral is a break down in social care but with no alternative to hospital admission this was the only previous option. The Health Authority has agreed funding for an additional four 'flexi-beds' at the Sir Alfred Jones Memorial Hospital on a pilot basis for three months as an additional resource for the ERT.

The Emergency Response Team can also offer support to patients seen in A and E. They are able to put in place 'resettlement programmes' over a 24 hour period. The need is predominantly for domicialary support but a follow up check visit by the nursing team is in place to ensure that nothing untoward has been missed. In addition Social Services have access to two emergency care beds which can be used in the short term to divert unnecessary admission. Current use runs at around 90 % occupancy.

In the first month that the service was introduced 8 calls were taken. Four months after its introduction this had risen to120 calls in a single month.

In addition Challenge Fund money was used to introduce a co-ordinator for elderly care with aims of improving screening programmes for over 75s, and acting as an inter-agency advocate. This initiative was initially set up as a trial using a controlled study design. Unfortunately the study design appeared to hamper the development without being sufficiently sensitive to the changes, during a time when the service was being developed. The scheme is no longer operational but the two remaining members of the team will become members of an Elderly Resource Team, building on their experiences of inter-agency working. Involvement of the wider community as well as health care workers in prevention and/or early detection of ill health is the key to the approach which will be taken. The whole systems 'San Diego' model[26], which strongly advocates this approach to facilitate multi agency working, is one which is being considered.

Contact details

Mrs P Bennett
Unit Leader – Intermediate Care
North Mersey Community Trust
Rathbone Hospital
Mill Lane
Liverpool
L13 2LP
Tel: 0151 250 4046

Mrs S Last
Continuing Care Manager
Liverpool Health Authority
Hamilton House
24 Pall Mall
Liverpool
L3 6AL
Tel: 0151 236 4747

[26] Elderly Health San Diego http://www.elderlyhelpofSandiego.org

Outlands Resource Centre
Plymouth

Purpose

Outlands is sited near the centre of Plymouth in a 1960's purpose built unit which originally offered residential accommodation, managed by social services, for 64 clients. Now the building houses:

- a 23 bedded rehabilitation unit for older people (which is the focus of this report)
- sixteen beds which are used for respite care
- an active day centre with places for up to 45 clients each week day and 16 on Saturdays and Sundays
- a further small day centre which is open five days a week for up to eight elderly people who are also mentally infirm.
- a carers support group, run jointly with social services

In addition they also house the incontinence laundry service for Plymouth, co ordinate meals on wheels and prepare food for the local disability unit throughout the week and meals on wheels at weekends.

Background and context

The rehabilitation unit (Outlands Resource Centre) was opened in 1992. The drive for its development came, not from a strategic overview of local need, but recognition that provision of residential care was steadily moving into the independent sector. If Outlands, which at that time was in urgent need of building update, was to survive it would have to review its place in the wider provision of services. Thus the changes were 'provider', rather than 'purchaser' driven.

Fortuitously this thinking coincided with a county wide review of residential care at a time when there were insufficient resources to meet the demand for residential accommodation, coupled with a backlog of people in acute care awaiting assessment and social services derived care packages. This led to generation of the idea of 'Community Care Support Centres' which would provide a specialist resource for multi professional assessment and rehabilitation for older people, develop such facilities in the independent sector and be a source of authoritative information. Outlands, however, was not designated as one of these resource centres so the team, faced with a risk of closure, looked to alternative strategies

A compounding factor came from the drive of the consultant geriatrician who was concerned with the pattern of care for older people. In his view there were times when an inappropriate 'crisis' admission to residential care was made which became irretrievable when, for example, that person's home had been either sold or re-let. His support in developing the plans for Outlands was significant.

Getting going

Collaboration between managers in the acute health care sector and the hospital social work team led to a specification of need driven by:

- changes in the NHS which were placing high demand on acute provider units for increased productivity
- the then newly introduced community care reforms. The often traumatic circumstances of patients admission meant that it was not feasible to undertake an accurate high quality assessment until late in the patients stay which could lead to considerable delay or inappropriate decision making in relation to discharge

The jointly agreed aim of this collaboration was:

> *'To gain practical experience of diverting people from residential care at the point of discharge from hospital, by providing a facility which would enable them to make well-judged decisions about the future level of support they would need.'*[27]

A joint steering group was set up at the outset of the Outlands project with two main functions which were 'twin packaged', namely to plan for the new service and concurrently to establish an evaluation strategy. Membership of the group included business managers, the lead consultant and physiotherapy and occupational therapy managers from the acute and community health trusts. Social services were represented by the Community District Team manager, the Outlands Unit manager and the Hospital Social Work Team manager.

The team were challenged not only with developing a new service but ensuring the safe and acceptable resettlement of many of the long standing Outlands residents. Considerable effort went into helping to re-house them and time was invested in supporting them and their families in finding alternative homes for their long term future. Ultimately all but 10 of the residents moved on to a new placement and, at a six monthly follow up visit, were found to have settled well. This was a time of high anxiety for the staff at Outlands who were uncertain about their own future. It was recognised that they too would need support through parting and grieving for clients for whom they had cared, in some instances, for many years. Helping in their resettlement gave them some opportunity to work through this process successfully.

Minimal funds (£4,500) from Social Services were invested in refurbishing Outlands and supplying

---

[27] Younger-Ross S, Lomax S, Cartwright M, Hamblin D *From Hospital to Home: the Outlands Project* Case Study 15 Plymouth Outlands

a rehabilitation kitchen on the top floor, intentionally away from the 'ethos' of residential care on the other floors of the building. Initially 10 beds, all in single rooms, were opened for a trail period of six months to clients with rehabilitation needs. Since then the number has increased to 23 beds.

What is on offer

Operational policies were developed for the unit from the outset. Referrals were made from the acute unit via the hospital social work team but the unit manager retained the right of refusal if he did not consider that the newly developed services at Outlands could meet the needs of a particular client.

Admission criteria included:

- clients would require no further inpatient medical treatment
- clients agreed to the transfer in full knowledge of the purpose and funding implications
- the care manager considered that the client could return home in a specified time
- nursing needs could be met by the Community District Nursing team
- clients were ready and eager to commence the rehabilitation programme
- clients were not confused or suffering from dementia
- clients were resident in the West Devon Social Services boundary
- clients would (usually) be aged 55 or above

In addition places were offered to clients who were motivated to go home. Referral sources for the period from 1st September to 31st December 1997, which reflect an overall trend, are given in figure eight and the age range in figure nine.

Figure eight – Referral sources September – December 1997

Referral Source	Number and percentage	
Orthopaedic	25	40%
Medical /General	20	32%
Care of the Elderly	10	16%
Accident and Emergency	3	5%
Rheumatology	1	2%
Surgical	3	5%
Total over four months	60	100%

Figure nine – Age Group

Age Group	Number and percentage	
Below 60	4	6%
60+	8	13%
70+	19	31%
80+	26	42%
90+	5	8%

An individualised programme of care, devised to prevent admission to residential care by substantially increasing levels of independence is offered to clients, the majority of whom spend six weeks in the unit. In exceptional circumstances, such as the need to find new accommodation, a stay may extend beyond this time frame but this is a rare occurrence.

Care programmes are based on care plans, developed by the social services care manager's assessment of need, who is the primary commissioner of the service. Within 36 hours of transfer a further assessment is made by the Outlands therapists in order to fine tune the care plan to match agreed client need with the services within the unit. This plan is then used as the basis for ongoing care. Continuity is provided by the care assistant key workers who are instrumental in supporting clients in regaining basic activity of living skills. Their work is managed with the backup of local guidelines.

At a mid point in the programme there is usually a further assessment coupled with a home visit which not only allows progress to be monitored but is also the point at which a home care package is planned for the future. Liaison with the district care manager is also initiated at this stage to help ensure a smooth transition back into the community. There is a follow-up discharge review at 2 and 5 weeks to ensure the safety and welfare of the client.

Staff profile and development

The staffing profile for the rehabilitation unit includes:

Social Services funded (some figures are approximate)

The Outlands unit manager	1 wte
Rehabilitation unit manager	1 wte
Care assessment officer	1.8 wte
Care assistants	12.6 wte
Domestic help	2.3 wte

Health funded

Physiotherapists	1 WTE
Occupational therapist	1 WTE

Access to speech therapy through health services.

Initial difficulty was experienced in gaining GP cover for patients who were not in their home 'patch'. Instead 1.5 hours of medical cover a week were funded separately by social services. There is also access to up to 10 hours of community nursing care each week. These figures are currently under review in the light of the new Partnership guidance.

Both the rehabilitation unit manager and the majority of care assistants were recruited internally from the team who had previously offered care to long term residential clients. High value was placed on their local 'knowledge and know-how'. The therapy staff developed an in-house training programme for the care assistants, the focus of which was to help them to move from a culture of dependence to one were independence was actively fostered. In addition there was some skill training in helping them to support clients in regaining skills in activities of living.

There is a high degree of stability in the Outlands team with minimal need for recruitment. Sickness levels are low and staff appear to be motivated by seeing people regain independence, a factor which they had not experienced previously when working with residential clients.

Funding

Funding for Outlands has been shared between health and social services from the outset, (see above) although it must be added that this example of interagency working was not easy to establish prior to joint commissioning. It is the view of the evaluation team that this development would have greatly assisted the Outlands project at the time it was established and that widening the collaboration to encompass housing and education agencies would also be of benefit.

A set contribution from clients was fixed at £48.50/week when the project was established bearing in mind that the majority of people who entered the programme were still maintaining their own homes. More recently the client contribution has been subject to means testing with an increase for some people up to £150/week. Unfortunately this appears to have had an impact on the way in which the service is used, with a decrease in length of stay at Outlands for some clients and a commensurate risk that the full impact of the rehabilitation programme cannot be achieved.

The whole charging policy for both social services driven rehabilitation and assessment will be the subject of review in the next year.

Evaluation

The service at Outlands has been evaluated from it inception, initially for a six month trial period and in a longer term follow up study. Of the 42 people who were admitted in the first six months following the opening of the unit all had previously been assessed as needing residential care. Following a six week period of rehabilitation all were discharged home. At the 5 year follow up there had been 22 deaths (after lengthy periods at home) and only 4 admissions to residential care[28]. Figure ten shows the overall discharge destination of patients over the six year period that the unit has been open.

---

[28] Younger-Ross S, Lomax T (1998) 'Outlands: Five Years On' *Managing Community Care* Vol 6 Issue 1 pp37-40

Figure ten – Discharge destination over a six year period

Number of admissions	1073
Home	845
Hospital	102
Residential and Nursing home	92
Other	20
Deceased	14

An estimate of cost savings based on the number of weeks a patient had spent at home following discharge less the cost of the six week programme was made. The evaluation team report an average saving of £15,200 per person and an aggregate saving of around £456,400 over a five year period.

The five year evaluation also followed up on the degree of domicilary support, which was minimal; the ongoing dependency which, for the small number of people on whom data was available appeared to be maintained or improved; and user views which, with one exception, were extremely positive.

Why it worked

Staff in the unit are clear that Outlands has been successful because of the 'common sense' approach they have taken which has included ensuring that:

- clients know what they are there for
- care has been taken to maintain a team spirit
- staff have been trusted to work well and in so doing have gained confidence
- admission criteria have been rigorously adhered to

They do not underestimate the complexity of establishing such a complex multi agency service but are convinced that the shared investment has also reaped shared benefits.

Where next

There are now plans to open other similar units across the county, and in particular ones which are able to accept patients directly from their homes. Plans are underway to develop a comprehensive data set of need, shared by health and social services, in order to assess the efficacy of different operational approaches to service delivery.

Contact Details

Mr Barry Luckman
Unit Manager
Outlands
Oates Road
Milehouse
Plymouth
PL2 3EJ

Tel: 01752 605704

Mr Peter Wells
Group Manager
City of Plymouth Social Services
Greville House
Buds Head Way
Crownhill
Plymouth
PL6 5ER
Tel: 01752 770540

Airedale NHS Trust Community Directorate Children's Service

Purpose of the service

Based on the premise that children should only be admitted to hospital if community resources cannot meet their needs, Airedale NHS Trust has developed a range of services as part of an integrated child health care strategy. To this end partnerships are fostered between families, health and social services, education and voluntary organisations in a concerted effort to ensure that children receive both preventative and curative services as near to home as possible.

Context

Airedale NHS Trust is a combined Trust serving a large, mixed urban and rural population covering more than 600 square miles. Hence access to central facilities can be time consuming and difficult. Within this context they have, over the past four years, developed a strategy which focuses on admission prevention where possible, and earlier transfer from acute settings. To this end their aim has been to develop a continuum of care encompassing primary, intermediate and acute facilities.

The Intermediate Care strategy complements other primary care services, aiming to provide local services for local populations. It is not seen as being dependant on buildings but on easy, speedy access to a range of procedures and treatments. The overall strategy has been a collaborative venture between health, social services and voluntary organisations, characterised by the development of an enhanced primary health and social care system, satellite out reach clinics, ready access to rehabilitation and therapy services and appropriate in-patient beds in the community. Four main principles have underpinned these moves, namely that care should be:

- effective and appropriate to the needs of individuals where risk is minimised
- available as near as possible to the person's home while remaining safe and effective
- provided as efficiently and effectively as possible
- enable equity of access to all within the resources available

This wider philosophy is reflected in the services which are offered to children, influenced by both local need and central policy. The services outlined below are targeted specifically at the interface between acute, primary and social care. In addition the Integrated Child Health Service includes a full range of acute and community nursing services including school nurses, care for those with learning disability, child and adolescent mental health services, district nursing and health visiting. There is also a Child Development Centre which provides a multi-disciplinary, multi-agency service to pre-school children with developmental difficulties and their families.

Getting Going

The range of children's services has been developed to ensure that skilled support is available in the community in order that children are only admitted to hospital when there is no other option; that they are discharged as soon as it is safe to do so; and parents feel able to mange their child's illness at home with support. Services include:

Children's Outreach Nurse – this services, which is acute care based, is concerned with discharge planning for children being transferred home who have ongoing nursing needs. Specialist nursing support is available for families and children at home in order to help them to 'bridge the gap' between home and hospital care. A key function is to ensure good liaison with the multidisciplinary team in primary, secondary and tertiary settings, in order to facilitate co ordination of the management of care and support early discharge from hospital. In addition there is an emphasis on admission prevention, sharing of expertise, and assurance of quality within an evidence based framework.

Referrals can be made to the service from acute and primary care, by doctors and nurses. They are directed to the specialist nurse but those children accepted into the service must be under the care of an acute care paediatrician.

Staffing – The service is provided by one WTE 'G' grade nurse who has general, children's and community qualifications. Arrangements have been made for cover in her absence through the Community Children's Nursing Service which demonstrates the way in which the services are integrated.

Patients – the range of patients cared for through this service includes those with needs related to IV antibiotic therapy, support for enteral feeding, tracheotomy care and anaphylaxis training for those at risk.

It is estimated that over a six month period twelve early discharges have been facilitated with an estimated saving of 157 bed days.

Funding – the main funding source for this service has been from the acute care budget.

Evaluation – An ongoing database has been established to ease record keeping and ensure availability of accurate up to date information. The service was audited in August 1998 confirming the needs addressed (as outlined above). The majority of referrals were received from outpatients or the children's ward. Liaison with many other health, education and social care providers was also evidenced and the service was sometimes used as an expert resource point.

In addition a Parent Satisfaction Survey was conducted in August 1998. There was a 32.5 % return rate with all respondents finding the service useful but with a call for more home visits. Positive comments were received in relation to improved communication with consultants and being able to stay at home.

Children's Home Nursing and Community Support Services – this service compliments the one outlined above but is community based. Currently a pilot service is being run which will potentially influence a wider community model. The aim of the service is to provide a home based service for the management and treatment of an agreed range of acute illnesses. Help is available to assist with discharge planning and assessment of care plans; prevention of admission or re admission; support to families including teaching them basic care skills; provision of palliative care, alongside support and advice to community nursing teams with a staff training provision.

Referrals are accepted from general practitioners and nurses as well as from the Children's Outreach Nurse. Referrals can be made directly into this service but most children are already well known to the hospital based paediatrician.

Staffing – the service was initially provided by a 0.5 WTE 'E' grade community paediatric nurse, based in a general practitioner's surgery. This has been increased to one WTE since October 1998.

Patients – the range of patient needs managed through this service is wide ranging including those related to IV drug therapy, redressing of surgical wounds or burns, monitoring of chronic conditions such as cardiac or renal problems, advice and support following orthopaedic and reconstructive surgery and palliative care.

It is estimated that over a six month period eight children were cared for who would otherwise have needed hospital admission, saving approximately 32 bed days. A further 40 children were cared for at home who would otherwise have needed to attend regularly at out patients department for dressings or blood tests.

Funding – original funding for this post came from the community budget with whole systems money being used to increase the establishment last October. It is hoped that this money will be recurring in the future but plans have yet to be confirmed.

Evaluation – this scheme is currently being subject to local evaluation using questionnaires to elicit parents views of the service, the impact that the community outreach nurse has had, and the percieved benefits to the child and family

Anecdotal evidence from the district nursing team and the acute hospital services suggests positive benefits include preventing the need for hospital attendance and providing skilled training and support to community teams and families.

Clockhouse

Clockhouse is a joint venture between health and social services that provides a range of services for children with ongoing health problems, which has been established to reduce their need for hospital admission. They are able to offer:

- after school care
- day care at weekends
- residential respite care (3 beds) on alternate weekends
- residential care for six weeks of the summer holidays
- a summer play scheme

In practice packages of care are very flexible and are arranged according to the needs of the individual children and their families.

Plans are currently underway for a jointly funded extension to facilities, in order to create a Health and Social Day Care Facility on site.

Staffing – Social Services were originally responsible for the Clockhouse site where two separate services were provided within the same accommodation, one from health and one from social services. Work has since been undertaken to integrate these two elements. All members of the team are managed by the Clockhouse Manager within the social services organisation. The team comprises:

a unit manager who has a professional background in social work
1 WTE 'E' grade nurse
O.8 WTE 'D' grade nurse
2.5 WTE 'A' grade care assistants

Therapy services are available through the support of peripatetic workers and additional support from the Child Development Centre social worker is also available.

The nurses are still employed by the Trust from whom they can receive professional support.

Patients/clients – many of the children who attend Clockhouse have severe disabilities and complex, sometimes life threatening, conditions. In consequence expert nursing is provided on a regular basis. Clinical conditions are wide ranging and include those with Cerebral Palsy, Batten's disease and Rhetts Syndrome. In some cases there is an anticipation that health will deteriorate over time with a commensurate increase in their demands for more complex health care. Individual packages of care are arranged according to need. While not attending Clockhouse the children are cared for at home or school.

The Clockhouse team have direct telephone contact with the paediatrician caring for each child should the need arise for urgent advice or should their condition deteriorate beyond the level which can be managed in the community.

Funding – Clockhouse was initially established on temporary Social Service funds. This funding has since been made recurrent. Health funding is provided for the nursing members of the team as well as for individual packages of care developed to meet specific family needs. Since 1997 there has been recurrent funding from the Health Authority for this aspect of the service.

Consultant access

An underlying principle behind the developments in Airedale is that there should be easy access to expert consultant paediatrician advice through either the community or acute care consultant. The most common approach is through telephone contact. Some outreach clinics are offered. Assessment can be undertaken in a range of different settings according to need.

Why has it worked?

The main reason behind the success of the integrated children's service is seen to be the joint nature of the venture which has allowed those involved to develop a seamless service. Parent involvement has been a critical factor in order that services truly match need. Issues which have been important to both users and providers of care have included:

- prevention of admission to hospital
- respite close to home
- the informal nature of the service
- the non institutional setting and approach to care

What next

The Trust is currently considering expansion of the services outlined above which will be influenced by both outcomes of the evaluation and resource allocation. In particular consideration is being given to the introduction of a specialist neonatal service with the aim of facilitating early discharge from hospital when this is in the best interest of the infant and family. In addition it is hoped that the number of beds at Clockhouse can be increased to 5 to meet the increasing need for this service. It is also hoped that there will be a dedicated therapy service and a play worker for Clockhouse. Partnership with families is seen as central to all these developments.

Contact names

Denise Arnott
Director of Inter-Agency Development
Community Division Headquarters
Coronation Hospital
Springs Lane
Ilkley
West Yorkshire
LS29 8TG
Tel: 01943 817370

Carole Donaldson
Locality Manager
The Health Centre
Oakworth Road
Keighley
West Yorkshire
BD21 1FA

Tel: 01535 295649

Part Three

Introduction

In this section of the report two outlines have been included of approaches to the development of a strategy which encompasses Intermediate Care as part of main line services. The first example summaries the way in which an acute Trust has developed a strategic plan for the future against a backdrop of inevitable change. This document is currently out for consultation.

The second example comes from a Health Authority who have completed a major consultation exercise, and agreed their strategic direction for the future. Operationalise of these plans will commence later this year.

Again, our purpose in including these reports is to raise discussion, in relation to local need.

City Hospital NHS Trust - Birmingham

A Strategic Approach

Background

City Hospital NHS Trust sees Intermediate Care as *"...an exciting opportunity to cultivate a diverse range of services, which are sensitive to patient need. Its introduction, however, heralds the beginning of an ambitious, challenging journey rather than a short term solution."*[29]

Faced with an inevitability that the pattern of health care in Birmingham would change, City Hospital NHS Trust have developed an alternative model of an 'Integrated Health System' for the future. Intermediate Care is one essential strand of this model, which has been developed after an exploration of local need, coupled with a review of different approaches to service delivery both at home and abroad. The aim of their proposal is to refashion the services which City Hospital provides within a collaborative relationship with other local service providers, based on the needs of the local population.

Multiple factors have led the team to seek an alternative approach to service delivery including:

- advanced medical technology allowing a move from in-patient to out-patient or day care treatment
- the local demography where the population has above average poverty, unemployment and ethnic minority communities
- a size of population which means that highly specialised services need to be centralised in order that sufficient numbers can be treated to maintain quality
- a focus on primary care in a setting where the vulnerability of General Practices, where one third of all principals will retire in the next decade, is recognised and the need to develop supportive complimentary services taken into account

An Integrated Health Care Network

City Hospital's vision is of an Integrated Health Services Network, with service provider partners from Primary Care Groups, Social Services, Local Authorities, Voluntary Organisations and other hospitals. They propose an agreement among the partners of clinical care pathways, encompassing the whole range of services required for specific illnesses or health related problems. They are suggesting a newly developed Ambulatory Care facility, based both at City Hospital and in Primary Care Centres (PCCs) and a range of Intermediate Care services. Figure eleven summarises the overall changes which they propose.

---

[29] City Hospital NHS Trust (1999) *The Way Forward – an integrated healthcare solution* Birmingham

Figure eleven – Proposed changes

The current process	The new process
Inpatient specialist treatment	Greater emphasis on ambulatory care in hospital and PCCs
Post acute care in hospital & inappropriate admissions	Intermediate care services & facilities
Hospital-based specialist diagnostics	Some diagnostics in PCCs with tele-links
Multiple diagnostics visits	One day diagnostics in Ambulatory Care Centre
Single hospital clinical departments	Integration of clinical service across hospitals
A&E department treating minor ailments	Large PCCs could have 'Urgent Care Centres' for minor ailments
Few non-medical specialists	Specialist non-medical staff
Specialty based departments	Multi specialty centres
Separate paper based medical records in hospital and Primary Care with varying treatment regimes	Electronic patient record shared with Primary Care and integrated care pathways
Treatment	Prevention and treatment

The model builds on the principles of a hub and spoke approach to care delivery, focusing on the entire continuum of health need, rather than just secondary health services. Where City Hospital does not have a large enough patient population to stand alone in specific specialties they aim to work together with other provider units. In some instances they may offer the 'hub' highly specialised services for their catchment group, returning patients to other sites for after care. In other specialties partners will offer the 'hub' service with City offering 'spoke' after care. Care for less complex cases within the service can also be offered in 'spoke' settings. For the less complex conditions seen most commonly, City Hospital aims to work collaboratively with Primary Care Centres who will provide decentralised care. This will leave room for the acute hospital to provide more complex treatment which requires advanced technology, at the central location.

This model would be facilitated by advanced technology to allow rapid access to diagnostic facilities and expert advice, decentralised clinics and services; a major increase in Ambulatory Care and Intermediate Care and the development of specialist roles among nurses and therapists to take services closer to people. Within this framework they see City Hospital at the forefront of undergraduate and post graduate teaching as it shifts to preparing practitioners to encompass working in Ambulatory and Intermediate Care settings as well as the more traditional environments. A key feature of this development will be the establishment of a Chair in Ambulatory Care.

The process

In order to develop their proposal City Hospital set up a series of working groups to explore aspects of service delivery including Acute Care, Ambulatory Care and Intermediate Care. These were seen within the overall context of a whole continuum of service provision encompassing self care at home, highly complex tertiary services, and Primary Care. The recommendations of these groups have been amalgamated in the current consultation document[30]. A brief summary of each groups recommendations has been included here in order to set the context of their suggestions for Intermediate Care. For the purposes of this document more detail of the exploratory process related to Intermediate Care have been included.

Acute care – this group's recommendations suggest a leaner tighter service underpinned by Ambulatory and Intermediate Care alongside shifts to community bases. They suggest concentrating the resources used to manage emergency admissions in one place, separate from

Figure 12 – Redesignation of bed numbers

Service	Bed numbers	
Short stay emergency	100	16%
Specialty	300	53%
Intermediate care and speciality rehab	200	31%
Total	**630**	**100**

(Existing compliment excluding certain categories e.g., ophthalmic services)

elective work. They envisage patients being grouped on disease condition lines. Recognition is given to changes in patient's dependency during acute and post-acute stages, with a need for much earlier access to rehabilitation. They suggest a re-designation of existing bed numbers could be as follows:

Ambulatory Care – this group undertook an assessment of current Ambulatory Practice through both an extensive literature review and a multidisciplinary visit to nine centres with a variety of sizes and configurations in the USA, and one in the UK. The model of Ambulatory Care they recommend encompasses comprehensive day care; outpatient services in a setting with a 'healing' environment; diagnostic suites for 'one stop assessment'; modular examination suites and a condition based clinical approach. They also recommend access to nursing and therapy led clinics, pharmaceutical services; audiology; infusion services; minor surgery and some alternative therapies.

State of the art communication and IT systems would be required to ensure the smooth running of

---

[30] City Hospital NHS Trust (1999) op cit

the services. In addition satellite services in PCCs are envisaged which may provide some aspects of care currently being offered in secondary settings. These would include imaging, minor surgery, out reach clinics and chronic disease management. Active 'Healthy Living Networks' in collaboration with PCCs all form part of the overall service.

Intermediate Care – this project group undertook an exploratory mapping exercise which provided:

- a snapshot of the national picture of Intermediate Care and an outline of the international perspective
- identification of the main groups or models of service provision seen in the literature, through personal networking and site visits
- a 'points prevalence' study to estimate the number of patients in the City Hospital NHS Trust and surrounding locality who may benefit by Intermediate Care at a single point in time

The tool which they developed for this work built on previous studies which had attempted to identify the need for an alternative range of services[31,32], encompassing the elements shown in Figure thirteen. Data were gathered from acute medical, surgical and elderly care wards and a local general practice. The classification was verified by the lead consultant for the patient group.

Figure thirteen - Key components of the assessment tool

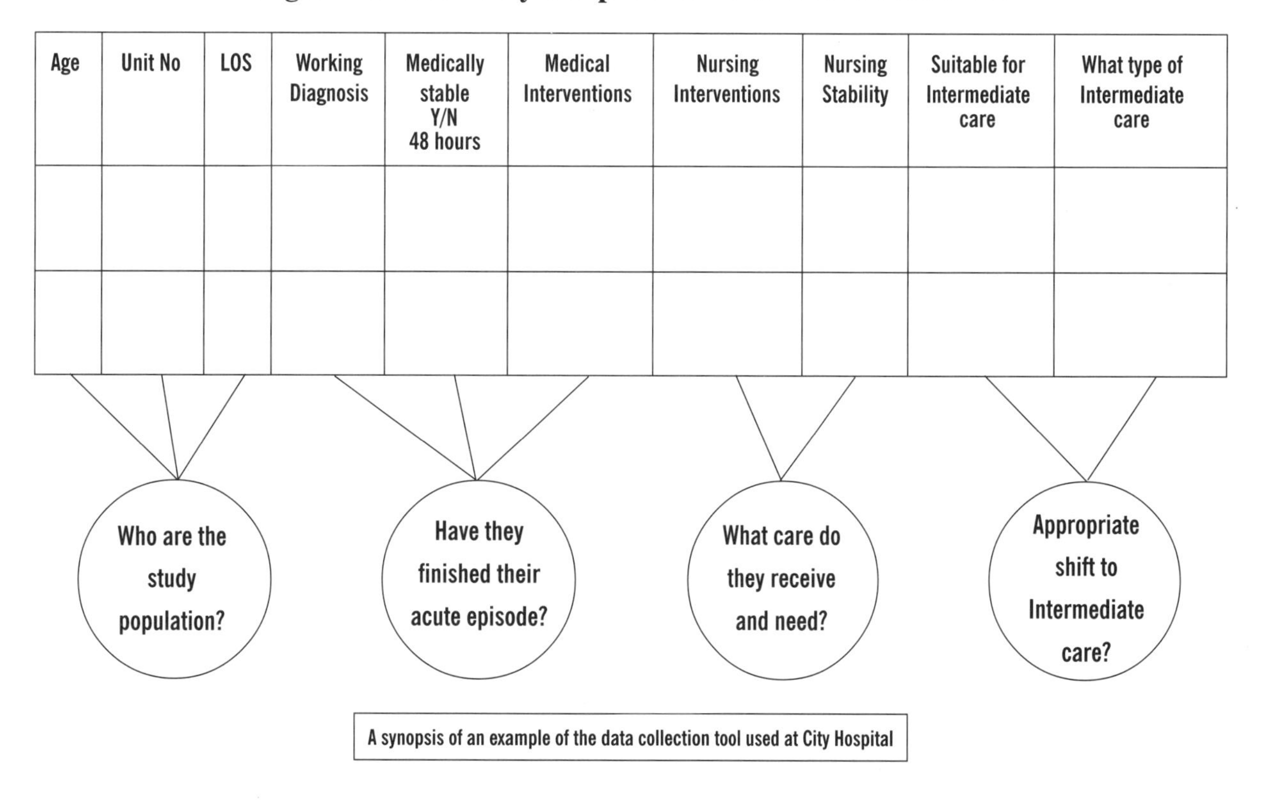

Age
Unit No
LOS
Working Diagnosis
Medically stable Y/N 48 hours
Medical Interventions
Nursing Interventions
Nursing Stability
Suitable for Intermediate care
What type of Intermediate care
Who are the study population?
Have they finished their acute episode?
What care do they receive and need?
Appropriate shift to Intermediate care?

A synopsis of an example of the data collection tool used at City Hospital

---

[31] Inglis A, Coast J, Frankel S (1996) Alternatives to Hospital Care: What are they and who should decide? *British Medical Journal* 312 162-6

[32] Victor C R, Khakoo A A (1994) Is hospital the right place? A survey of 'inappropriate' admissions to an inner London NHS Trust Journal of Public Health Medicine Vol 16 no 3 286-290

[33] City Hospital HNS Trust (1999)

In total 441 patients were assessed in the study. Initial analysis suggests that 25% of the patients occupying acute beds could be cared for in an Intermediate Care setting with a further 17% awaiting residential or nursing home care. The team suggest that " ...these are early results and are considered to be conservative."[33]

The preferred options for care suggested by the study are for nurse-led wards (44%), Hospital at Home (27%) and Step down facilities (29%). These findings have been coupled with the views of the Acute Group project team to suggest that there is a current need which could be meet by:

Figure fourteen - Movement of patients across a continuum of care incorporating Intermediate Care

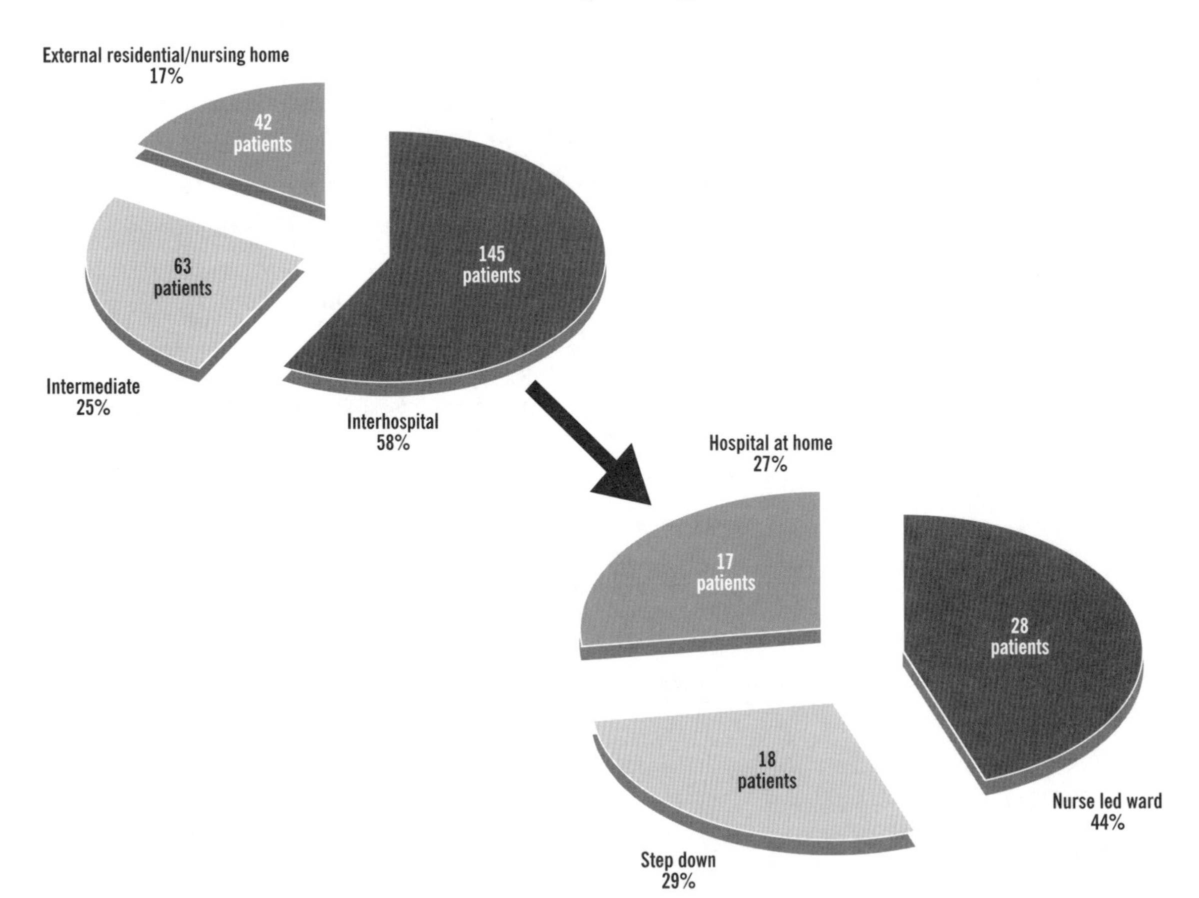

- 45 beds in Nurse Led Units
- 23 Hospital at Home places
- 27 places in step down facilities
- A rapid response team (size yet to be determined)

As part of their work this group also undertook a communications exercise in order to explain the remit they had been given, to respond to any queries and to elicit the views of others. Two events were held, one internal to City Hospital and one to a wider audience across Birmingham with a potential interest in the initiative. This included community based colleagues, health authority personnel, social services, and user representation. In addition they sort the advice of an external consultant with expertise in this approach to service delivery.

A summary of the conclusions this group drew suggests that it would not be possible to develop an integrated model without Intermediate Care services, but that the need is not always recognised

until viable options are offered as alternatives to current service. They recommend replication of the points prevalence study. Other implications are that:

- there are significant workforce issues to be addressed at an early stage in order to ensure that the right people with appropriate skills are recruited and/or trained prior to the introduction of new services
- joint inter-agency working is essential to success
- multi- professional work which minimises overlap of function and maximises the skills of all team members is critical
- the learning needs of patients and carers in relation to Intermediate Care must be addressed

The Future

City Hospital have recently published a report of their suggested strategy with three stated objectives:

- to share ideas and seek the views of members of the community whom they serve
- to act as a catalyst for the Trust's organisational and professional development activities
- as the backdrop to the preparation of a Strategic Outline Case for future developments

This report will be widely circulated in order to elicit maximum feedback prior to making formal proposals for the future within their Strategic Outline Case.

Contact

David Roberts
Director of Corporate Affairs
City Hospital NHS Trust
Dudley Road
Birmingham
B18 7QH
Tel: 0121 507 4419

Catherine Elcoat
Director of Nursing Practice
City Hospital NHS Trust
Dudley Road
Birmingham
B18 7QH
Tel: 0121 507 4795

East Norfolk Health Authority

Intermediate Services Strategy

Background

East Norfolk HA interprets *intermediate services* as meaning services which sit between those offered routinely by a family doctor and his or her team, and those available in a DGH. This definition goes beyond the normal scope of *Intermediate Care* (those services which facilitate the transition from an acute care setting to home (or help to divert admission to an acute care setting) by improving health through timely therapeutic intervention) to include continuing and palliative care.

East Norfolk HA faces a significant problem, in that people living within its borders currently do not enjoy equal access to "intermediate services" – for example, there are few community-based beds in Norwich. Many people have to travel outside their area for in-patient care in a community bed and only 27 out of 86 GP practices can refer patients directly to such beds. At present therapy staff work across a variety of locations with a mix of patients and community hospitals in the area, providing a range of services to patients with a variety of health needs. There is no standard practice.

The Health Authority's new intermediate services strategy separates out three core elements of "intermediate" care: rehabilitation, community-based beds and day treatment and therapy - elements which in many cases are currently delivered in the same setting. The strategy is designed to ensure more focused care for patients to meet their particular needs, at the right time and in the right place to maximise recovery. It will also create a high-quality, flexible pattern of care that can respond to the changing needs of users and take full advantage of new developments. Although the number of community beds will fall from 458 to 342, many of these beds are not currently used, some are occupied by long-stay residents and occupancy rates average only 71%. The new intermediate services strategy anticipates improving community bed occupancy rates to at least 85%.

The map in Figure fifteen shows the current distribution of community hospitals within East Norfolk Health Authority. Nearly all of these are located in the north and west of the Health Authority. A map showing the proposed new pattern of services is shown in Figure sixteen.

Process

In summer 1997, the HA set up a public involvement project to develop both quantitative and qualitative information about people's understanding of intermediate services and the values they placed on having those services close to home. This was repeated with GPs, "informed"

Figure fifteen - current distribution of community hospitals within East Norfolk Health Authority

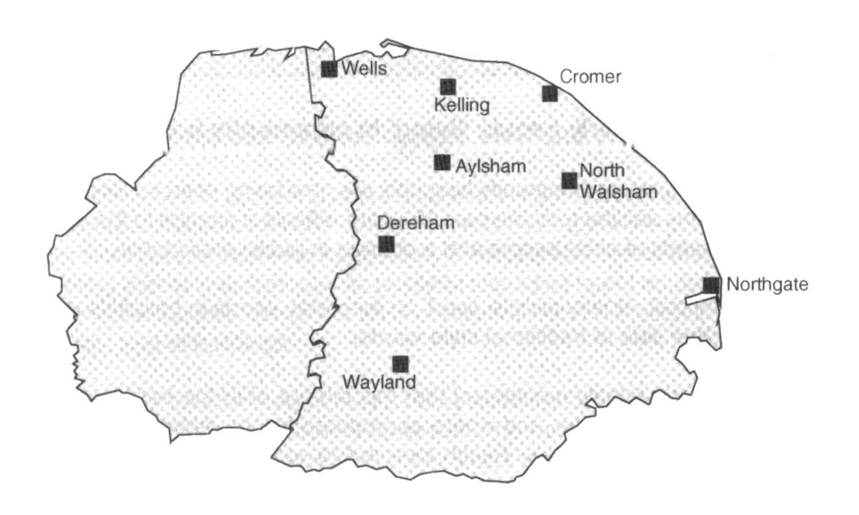

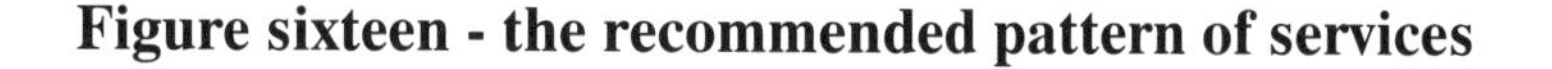

Figure sixteen - the recommended pattern of services

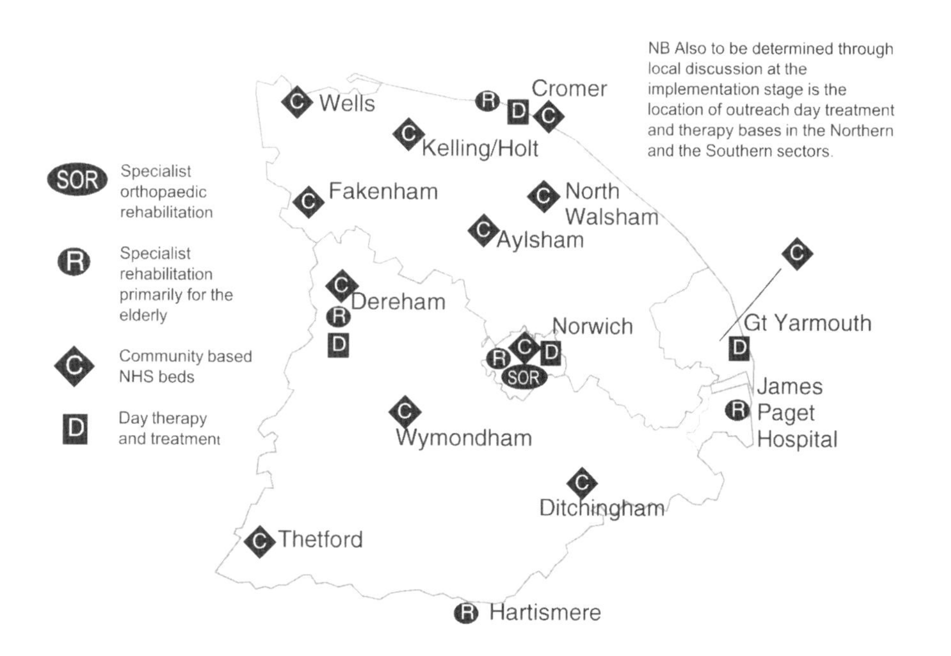

stakeholders and voluntary sector representatives. The findings of this work were then used to inform the next stage of the process, and to provide a framework for communication.

Key messages to come out of the public involvement exercise included:

- general difficulty understanding the whole concept of what is meant by "intermediate services"; and
- great allegiance to buildings and the need for more pro-active communication about the enormous amount of NHS care that does not rely on a building or an NHS bed for its delivery.

The Health Authority then divided East Norfolk into four sectors. Each sector drew together a range of representatives, including GPs, nurses, therapists, CHC representatives, Trust and HA staff, to draw up intermediate service proposals for their sector based on their local knowledge and understanding of patients needs. Each sector met at least twice to develop its proposals, drawing on localised information from a toolkit. This included population profiles, activity data, financial information, public opinions, morbidity and mortality information. While the sector groups were working, the HA distributed 300,000 copies of a newspaper explaining the process and what it meant by intermediate services. Local CHCs held public meetings to talk about what was happening and seek local views to feed into the sectors.

Public Consultation

5,000 copies of a draft strategy "Facing the Future: Ensuring NHS Care that Counts" setting out far reaching changes in the tier of Intermediate Care health services were published in July 1998, and circulated for a three months public consultation period. 50,000 copies of a summary of the strategy (including a pro-forma response) were also published, and the Health Authority held a series of 12 high-profile, well-attended public meetings. In addition many presentations, and question and answer sessions, were held with district councils, voluntary organisations, the CHCs and other representative groups. In all about 1400 responses were received and over 3000 people attended public meetings.

During the consultation it became apparent that two key issues dominating discussions were:

- access to the Health Authority's proposed locations for services
- the number of beds being proposed for this intermediate sector

The Health Authority commissioned independent research on both these issues and published the findings before a decision about the future was made. This research concluded that overall access would be improved if there was a fourth rehabilitation centre and recommended that bed numbers should be increased from the Health Authority's original proposal of 316 to 342 in discussion with Primary Care Groups. There would be a choice of more beds or increased community services. The recommendations were accepted.

Following the consultation process some changes were made to the proposed pattern of services to respond to views and concerns raised and to strengthen the overall pattern of care.

A full analysis of all the responses received during the consultation process was made available to members and anyone else who wanted it. Final decisions were taken at a meeting of the Health Authority held in public at which all those attending had the opportunity to comment and ask questions.

The Agreed Intermediate Services Strategy

The main elements of the new pattern of intermediate care services will be as follows:

- a specialist orthopaedic rehabilitation service for patients who have undergone joint replacements at the Norfolk and Norwich hospital
- four specialist rehabilitation centres for older people at Norwich (new), Cromer (new), Dereham and James Paget Hospital(Great Yarmouth), staffed by nurses, doctors, therapists, and social workers
- community based beds at twelve sites throughout East Norfolk
- a network of four new day treatment and therapy centres (Norwich, Cromer, Dereham, Great Yarmouth) with satellite outreach bases in Northern and Southern Norfolk. The main centres will be sited alongside the specialist rehabilitation centres. These centres will provide a base from which people can receive therapy services from health professionals (nurses, physiotherapists, occupational and speech and language therapists, chiropodists and dieticians). They will also provide a base for some new clinics, e.g. cardiac rehabilitation, back pain and rapid access assessment for older people (allowing GPs to arrange a number of tests and investigations quickly and closer to home). Additional day treatment and therapy in the more rural areas will be provided from primary care settings.

Consequences of the Strategy

The recommendations agreed by the Health Authority means that there will be changes to existing NHS community hospitals and other health care facilities. Of the 8 community hospitals within East Norfolk HA, one will close (Wayland Hospital in Attleborough). The other seven community hospitals are currently located in towns where the HA has identified a need for community-based beds and other services. The next stage of implementing the strategy will be to decide (through local consultation) the best site for these beds and other services in those towns. There will be a full option appraisal of possible sites and in each of the cases the community hospital site will automatically be considered. If, as a result of this option appraisal, the community hospital site is felt to be the best location for local people, there could be substantial change to the site as it currently exists

The benefits of the strategy include:

- eight new facilities for people in East Norfolk including three new centres of excellence for rehabilitation primarily for older people, a new centre with community-based NHS beds in Norwich and four new day treatment and therapy centres
- the development of consistent quality of NHS services across the area
- enhanced professional development and training for staff
- a more logical, flexible, better co-ordinated pattern of service which fits NHS services round patients, rather than trying to fit patients into current services

- dedicated rehabilitation care in a range of new or redeveloped facilities allowing specialist staff to work together more effectively in teams
- more therapy staff working with family doctors as part of their teams; and
- better access – many people will no longer have to travel out of their area to use community-based NHS beds.

Next Steps

The Health Authority is now moving on to the next stage – the publication of the implementation plan. There will be an option appraisal for each element of the strategy in each sector. Key issues to decide will include: site selection, staffing and training requirements, detailed arrangements for new elements of care (e.g. the specialist rehabilitation service, day treatment and therapy) and the time-tabling of the changes to maintain the quality of existing services while developing new style services. There will be public consultation on the option appraisal. The HA will continue to involve a wide range of people in the implementation process including consultants, family doctors, representatives from the CHC, as well as NHS Trusts, Norfolk Social Services and HA planners.

Once agreed the timetable for the changes will be published so that people can see when changes in their particular area will be taking place. It is hoped to start implementation in autumn 1999 with changes happening over the following three years. There is flexibility for bed numbers to rise as high as 361 if, at the implementation stage, all PCGs chose to opt for more NHS community beds in preference to additional community resources.

Contacts

Vanessa Wood
Intermediate Services Project Manager
Norfolk Health Authority
St Andrews
North Side
St Andrews Business Park
Thorpe St Andrews
Norwich NR7 0HT
Tel: 01603 300600

Debbie Bartlett
Norfolk HA Public Affairs
Norfolk Health Authority
St Andrews House
North Side
St Andrews Business Park
Thorpe St Andrews
Norwich NR7 0HT
Tel: 01603 300600

Part Four

Introducing Intermediate care – Short and long term implications

If there was a single way of describing the developments in this report it would be the common sense and simplicity which characterises the services, but the complexity of introducing them. On the whole their development has been needs driven, based at one end on a percieved gap in service provision, and at the other end on an opportunity to fill that deficit, usually owing to access to opportunistic funding, or excessive pressure elsewhere in the system. They are, universally, a demonstration of the commitment and energy of the teams concerned who have been prepared to look for creative alternatives to the traditional patterns of service provision. The services themselves are not dependent on sophisticated environments. Indeed one comment was that "...we could take this service and run it anywhere."[34] Rather, they are based on a clear vision of need, a matching provision of care and the confidence to proceed.

Yet as the contributors have told their tales it is evident that bringing about change, in the context of Intermediate Care, is as complex and difficult as in any new situation. While there are shared drivers there are also shared inhibitors to the developments. In this section some of those drivers and inhibitors are highlighted alongside the wider long term implications for service development policy, and education.

Practical steps in implementation

As data has been gathered for this report recurring themes from each of the contributors have become evident. They come as no surprise, yet are worth noting for future developments, in order that strategies can be developed to enhance the driving forces and minimise the effects of the inhibitors.

Time to get going – The time which it takes to develop a new service, to ensure that others know of its existence, and to assess its efficacy, is usually underestimated, which can led to a dilemma. On the one hand, if a window of opportunity arises, such as short term funding, there is a drive to explore a new service provision quickly. On the other hand, short term funding can frustrate a strategic, whole systems approach to service provision. Yet if new services are developed without adequate planning and preparation there is a high risk that they will fail. The ground work behind their introduction is critical to success, in terms of both staff development and communication strategies, if competence of the practitioners and confidence in the service is to be assured.

Time impacts on a myriad of other factors too. Referral to any new service may be slow in the early

---

[34] Homerton Hospital p 29

days, which will hinder the ability to recognise the knock on effect in other parts of the organisation initially. Thus if insufficient time is allowed for a service to become fully established, a false picture can be gained of its potential value. In the same way it takes time for the practitioners involved to recognise the degree of complexity they can manage in relation to the needs of the patients they accept into their care. A recurring pattern in these developments can be recognised where the level of patient need which can, for example, be managed in the community or in a nurse-led facility, gradually increases as confidence is gained by those providing the service and those referring to it. Hence if an assessment of use is made too early in the introduction of new services a false picture may emerge.

Staffing and recruitment – one of the factors which has underpinned the development of Intermediate Care services is the degree of commitment of the staff. Hence an assurance that the right person is doing the right work in the right place becomes critical. The way in which staff recruitment and development has been dealt with has varied from site to site but remains a significant issue. Evaluation of the schemes supported by Winter Pressures funding suggests that they have been slow to start owing to recruitment problems, particularly of therapy staff. With the limited supply of some staff groups it is helpful to anticipate the possibility of recruitment difficulties and consider how they may be countered. Many schemes have employed agency staff but this approach reinforces the short term nature of the schemes themselves and is not conducive to effecting real change in service provision.

There is a case to be made for investing in staff who are already working locally, who have knowledge of local provision and who are interested in expanding and developing their roles. In this instance there are excellent examples of multi professional in-house development programmes. However it must be stressed that without the introduction of such programmes both staff and patients are put at risk and the 'Sitting next Aunt Nelly' approach to learning is not an acceptable option.

In other situations there has been a need for a strong managerial stance, when staff who have become familiar with a traditional way of working are either unwilling or unable to change their patterns of behaviour. If such problems are not addressed then any new project can be put at risk. However, early recognition of this potential difficulty, use of good redeployment practices and involvement of relevant unions sooner rather than later, have all been found to be helpful. It must be added, however, that these issues do take time to handle.

Once units have been established another picture frequently emerges. The opportunity for people from all disciplines to undertake work which they find challenging and fulfilling appears to have a knock on effect on staff morale. Teams commonly report a reduction in sickness levels[35], increased stability in post[36] and no difficulty in recruitment[37]. Even in areas where there are significant

---

[35] Cass Ward – Homerton Hospital p 29
[36] Outlands resource centre p 41
[37] Sir Alfred Jones Memorial Hospital p 35

recruitment problems it has been suggested that the local community quickly learns that '...these jobs are good' and there are examples of one satisfied post holder recruiting other family members to the service[38].

These patterns fit well with descriptions of so-called Magnet Hospitals[39] in the USA where a common knowledge of the culture of the unit attracted able staff which, in turn, had a positive effect on quality of care.

Sustainability and roll out – an ongoing concern for many of the initiatives is how they will be sustained in both the short and long term future. Many are supported by short term funding which can create uncertainty in relation to security of jobs, opportunity for development and commitment to long term planning. Short term funding is also problematic in that it may stimulate demand for services which, when the funding runs out, no longer have the capacity to respond to need. Unless the agencies involved have the will and resources to commit to the continued delivery of such services then short term provision can prove frustrating, not least for patients who have come to expect them. This highlights the urgent need to bring together operational and strategic thinking in order that the position of innovation and its inter relation with other parts of the organisation can be explored.

Linked to this is a concern about long term leadership. Examples can be found where innovations have collapsed when the 'hero innovator' leader has moved on. Alternatively there are excellent examples where there has been very active succession planning with consideration of how both team members and leaders can be prepared for the future. Success, it should be stressed, has been marked by proactive management.

Many of the initiatives which have been described here are fairly small and their development has been strongly influenced by local contextual issues. Questions have been raised about the manner in which they can now be 'rolled out' to meet the needs of a wider population. That there should be equity of access to Intermediate Care across geographical patches is an important consideration. However, a contributing factor to the success of the pilot studies has been the flexible way in which they have been able to respond to, and build on, local needs and resources. Thus a concern has been expressed that, in trying to directly duplicate elsewhere, sensitivity to local need would be lost. This does not mean that the lessons learned cannot be built on, and that there can be some time-saving in expanding current Intermediate Care programmes. But the enormity of the cultural change from a service which is driven by the management of disease to one which focuses on enhancement of self care, rehabilitation and prevention of deterioration is often underestimated and must be dealt with at a local level if the quality of care is to be maintained.

Local learning seems to be a hallmark of these initiatives. There is no blue print for Intermediate

---

[38] Bedford and Shires
[39] Buchan J (1997) Magnet Hospitals: what's the attraction? *Nursing Standard* 12 (7) 22-25

Care – nor can there be since everyone is at a different starting point. Successful schemes are those which recognise a gap in service provision locally and plug that gap, or which offer a better alternative to current services. It is likely that for any given local health economy, a range of Intermediate Care services will be needed in order to ensure that they are responsive to the needs of patients. However, the detail of local provision must be determined by local needs and resources with new developments linked together to make a strategic, coherent whole.

Evaluation – that there is a need for sound evaluation is self evident but its execution is complex. Firstly there is a concern about timing. It has already been suggested that the introduction of any new service of this nature is a fluid process which changes over time as confidence and understanding of the service increases. Thus if data are collected at too early a point in the development they will not give a true reflection of the shape and efficacy of the service at a later stage. However there is an urgent need for iterative feedback from evaluation for service planners and providers in order to influence future service provision and professional development within a framework which considers health gains and outcomes.

The experience of those who have undertaken formal evaluation is that care must be taken to account for this fluidity in service development, especially when comparisons are being made of one service with another, but also with 'before and after' designs. These issues are dealt with in more detail elsewhere[40]. Suffice to say here that it is important to gather both process and outcome data in order to gain a complete picture of the developments and to note that timing of data collection in relation to the study design will have a significant impact.

Workload – the shifting of workload from one section of the service to another is a further factor for consideration. In relation to organisations it has been interesting to note that the drive for Intermediate Care services has arisen from acute, primary and social care settings and has been related to need, rather than age, or a disease related clinical speciality. This could suggest that there is a need to review the current manner in which services are 'packaged'. While it is hoped that the move to increase working partnerships[41] will break down some of the barriers, this has undoubtedly been problematic in the past.

Concern has been expressed about shifts in workload for the groups concerned, with related anxieties about whether the resources will follow the need. Thus as more care is moved into the community some general practitioners have raised questions about whether the cover offered should be a part of General Medical Services or be subsumed under the alternative model of Personal Medical Services. Questions have also been raised about whether there should be a dedicated Intermediate Care team for community based services or whether they should be subsumed into current community care services with a commensurate increase in the overall

---

[40] Steiner A, Vaughan B, Hanford L (1998) *Intermediate Care: Approaches to Evaluation* London King's Fund

[41] Department of Health (1998) *Partnership in Action: new opportunities for Joint Working Between Health and Social Services* London DoH

workload. Examples can be found of both approaches which have worked successfully. The common denominator is the need to monitor workload and ensure that the good will of practitioners is not abused.

Shifts in responsibility – it is not only workload which is shifting but also the responsibility for care. Patients are going home at an earlier stage in their clinical course or being offered care at home or in non acute settings which would previously have been hospital based. It is critical that the move in responsibility for both medical and other care is carefully managed and channels of communication between practitioners which are easy to access are assured. Of utmost importance is that this issue is recognised, although the solutions are varied. There are for example some schemes where the acute care medical team have retained clinical responsibility for patients being cared for at home, with the direct care givers (usually, but not always, the community nurses) being given authority to instigate re admission if necessary. It should be noted that it has seldom been necessary to exercise such authority.

An alternative model is one-to-one communication between the primary and acute care medical staff prior to patient transfer, with authority vested in the community staff not to accept a transfer if they consider that the care needs are too complex for them to be managed outwith the acute hospital setting. In this way some control can be retained over the type of patient need for which the Intermediate Care team take responsibility, giving them a greater feeling of autonomy.

There is a further shift in responsibility in some of the Intermediate Care services which is occurring between the occupational groups concerned. Again there are differing views. One perspective is a strong view that access to care should always be monitored through expert medical assessment. Such arguments can be persuasive. However there is a growing recognition that some of the rehabilitative and nurturing needs of many patients are more appropriately managed by nurses and therapists. Hence there is a need for them to be given the authority to manage care which is commensurate with their often extensive level of training, knowledge and skills. The question is how the interface between expert medical assessment and ongoing responsibility for rehabilitative care can be managed in order to ensure equity, in terms of service provision for all involved, while respecting the individual autonomy of practitioners. Team work is at the heart of Intermediate Care with effective multi-professional working relations which emphasis the part each team member has to play in a non hierachial way.

Shared learning has offered one solution to this dilemma where teams have, over time, learned more about the skills of colleagues. Time has helped those involved to gain confidence in the ability of others and reduce anxiety that patients will be put at risk. Open telephone lines for consultation have been found helpful, as have assurances of quick and easy access to specialist services should the need arise. Thus, provided that there can be a smooth flow of both information and, if needs be, of patients, between the different sectors these difficulties can be minimised.

Cross skilling – one of the characteristics of Intermediate Care units is a degree of cross skilling between the different occupational groups and specialties. There is evidence of the generic training of care assistants in community or social services settings, enabling them to support the work of both nurses and therapists. Most schemes have been established locally and are frequently run jointly by therapists and nurses.[42, 43]. At this level the schemes have been well received by both the professional groups and the care assistants, allowing them to offer more rounded services and breaking down some of the more traditional boundaries that have developed between the different occupational groups.

Such skill sharing is not confined to the development of care assistants and there are examples where nurses, therapists and doctors have also shared skills[44]. In this way, while not purporting to be expert in the unique contributions of each of the occupational groups, a more seamless services can be provided to patients and delay in an holistic first level assessment of need can be avoided. Equally if more people are trained to do more work a more intensive service can be provided for patients.

Sadly it must be noted that while these schemes have been very successful at an operational level there has been some resistance expressed by others who have not been directly involved, with concern about the uniqueness of each group's work being lost as boundaries become more blurred. Such anxieties need careful handling in order that colleagues are not alienated, but the skills of the local work force are best matched to patient need rather than professional pride.

Escalating demands – a word of warning was offered by several of those involved in relation to clarity of admission criteria. As with many other issues a continuum of view can be identified. At one end is the need to be flexible, not only in order to maintain good working relations with those who refer into Intermediate Care, but also to ensure that options are left open to guarantee that best use is made of the developing skills of the team. At the other end of this continuum is a fear that, unless there is rigid adherence to admission and discharge criteria the system will be open to abuse, inappropriate referrals will be made and any evaluation of outcomes will become distorted.

It must be stressed that, as services have developed over time and the competence and confidence of the practitioners has grown, there has been a shift in referral patterns to accommodate people with greater degrees of need. In itself this has been a continuing challenge for the clinical teams as they have been able to widen the range of care which they feel able to offer. There has, however, also been an ongoing need to publicise Intermediate Care as those responsible for referral, albeit through acute care, accident and emergency services or community care, change jobs and new staff are unfamiliar with the nature of the services.

---

[42] Outlands resource centre p 41

[43] Sir Alfred Jones Memorial Hospital p 35

[44] Ealing Intermediate Care Services p 10

Discussion – Future Implications

From the degree of activity in the field of Intermediate Care it would seem that such services are here to stay. Indeed any future health economy will need to encompass them in combination with other services in order to ensure delivery of seamless care, to meet local demands and make best use of limited resources. Currently, however, provision is patchy, funding is opportunistic and staff development and training largely dependent on local effort without, in many cases support from either the Royal Colleges or the educational institutions. Successful implementation on a wider front will almost certainly need to be considered from a whole systems perspective as the cross boundary and multi-agency nature of the work becomes more evident and specific question are raised in relation to longer term consequences. To date many of the innovations have been made possible through local endeavour. Now is the time to consider wider implications.

The Context and Culture of Change

The development of Intermediate Care comes at a time when the whole health care system is subject to change, as the impact of both internal and external forces is felt. Technology has already changed the face of many aspects of service including diagnostic techniques, surgery and pharmacological treatments. Communication systems have opened up new options for tele-medicine and telecare, as well as providing ways in which patients and clients can access health-related information directly. Workforce profiles are changing with a predicted short fall of general practitioners over the next ten years, an ongoing requirement to reduce the hours worked by junior doctors, a current shortfall of nurses and therapists and a proliferation of new roles. If the shifts in policy to a health service which is closer to the people, community based, with a public health and health promotion emphasis, are to be matched in practice then the need for change is great. At the same time, as the impact of clinical governance is felt, professionals and managers are rightly being held to account for equity of access and appropriateness of care. It is critical that there are local and national endeavours to support these changes.

To date the way in which developments have been introduced in health care has, it can be argued, been largely based on increasing specialisation in a highly reductionist way. As expertise has grown, small, highly skilled teams have achieved unthought of ways of managing complex health care problems, the benefits of which are self-evident. However, in a resource limited service, caring for an ageing population, with the advantage of options which are now possible through the wise use of technology, there is an imperative to seek alternative options, taking account of whole systems approaches, with the commensurate attention to multi-agency and multi-professional working. It is within this wider context that the development of Intermediate Care must be placed.

Practice and Culture – The influence of differing cultures of practice is a further compounding factor to consider. Why, for example, are patients in one setting referred to hospital while those with similar needs but in different settings are not? Patterns of referral vary widely throughout the country with concurrent variations in the manner in which local risk management is handled, perhaps linked to local variations in confidence, competence and communication systems. Patterns of service provision also vary and while social admissions are well recognised, the degree to which they occur is geographically inconsistent, in line with an inconsistency in availability of alternative options and approaches to practice. The demands of some families and patients for packages of care which may or may not be appropriate to need, but which they have come to expect as their rights, are also a key variant in creating differences in the manner in which care is offered.

The implications of this are apparent for both providers and receivers of care. Public expectation, fuelled by both the media and the more traditional paternalistic attitude of health care workers has, in the past, led to an unquestioning compliance among some service users. Alternatively, others may make demands for access to services which are not always available locally, may not yet be evidence based or may not meet clinical need. It is clear that if the nature or pattern of health care services are to change then there will need to be a major public relations exercise in helping people to learn how to use them to best effect, as well as a change in the relationship between care givers and recipients of care.

Already there is some suggestion that patients have a preference for services which facilitate independence[45], a philosophy which is in line with that of Intermediate Care. Thus a question must be raised about whether Intermediate Care is giving patients what they want - and soft evidence would suggest that it is.

Partnership in Care – The impact of partnership relationships on health professionals and the manner in which they work is also worthy of consideration. The rhetoric of moving to partnership models of practice should not be underestimated, nor the requirement of continuing professional education if it is to become a reality. It can be argued that to ask practitioners to change a life time way of working without investing in an infrastructure to support that change is likely to fail. Yet, as there is external pressure from policy makers for partnerships with patients[46], and an explosion of access to information for service users and providers alike, there is an inevitable knock on effect in working relationships of service users and providers. The complexity of these relationships is not uncommonly denied even though there is increasing evidence of lack of understanding and mixed messages between those who provide and those who use health care. Thus there is a particular concern because this need can go unrecognised.

Partnerships in care are not limited to relationships between health professionals and patients but are also concerned with inter-agency and inter-professional work[47]. Both forms of partnership are inherent principles which underpin Intermediate Care, which require proactive handling. There is

---

[45] Nuffield/University of Liverpool (1998) *Evaluation of the Implementation of the Continuoing Health Care Guidance*

[46] NHS Executive (1996) *Patient Partnership: Building a Collaborative Strategy* Leeds NHS Executive

[47] Department of Health (1998) *Partnership in Action: New Opportunities for Joint Working Between Health and Social Services* London DoH

an urgent need for greater understanding of the different cultures and philosophies of care in different sectors of the system alongside consideration of the pre- and post registration implications for professional education.

Role boundaries and professional education – A further major issue for debate, which has significant consequences for the future development of Intermediate Care, relates to role boundaries and professional education. Currently local programmes have been developed to help the people involved in service provision, whether they be doctors, therapists, nurses or generic support workers, to develop the requisite clinical and organisational skills necessary to offer effective care. Their efforts are to be applauded and there are many excellent examples of good practice. However this does raise several issues of concern.

Firstly there is huge duplication of effort as each new team develops an internal programme with or without external validation. Secondly there is a concern that both practitioners and patients could be vulnerable unless there are agreed baseline standards for safe practice, a concern which can directly be related to the current drive for National Service Frameworks[48]. Thirdly there is a concern about effective use of resources, raising questions about how better use can be made of a workforce which is currently under pressure. A case can be made, not only that there is some duplication of function, but that there are some sectors of the workforce who are over prepared for the level of responsibility which they have traditionally taken. Yet they find it difficult within the current system to make best use of their skills[49]. Thus there are some nurses and therapists who are qualified to Masters or doctoral level but who are restricted in the degree of autonomy with which they can practice within the current system.

The fourth issue is that, while there is wide discussion about substitution of roles in health care, most frequently concerning doctors and nurses, the roles developing in Intermediate Care do not always follow this path. Instead they combine some of the skills of one or more traditional roles in a way which is specific to the need of the patient group but blurs traditional role boundaries. Thus instead of substitution, an enhanced role has emerged in relation to the provision of more seamless care for the patient.

Finally a question must be raised about the way in which our current workforce is prepared, which is basically separatist in nature, emphasising differences rather than shared learning needs. It may be timely to reconsider professional education in relation to the changing health needs of the population, alterations in service delivery and a shift in balance between curative, preventative and rehabilitative aspects of care. While consideration of, for example a generic entry to health care, is not well received in many quarters since the essence of the different occupational groups may be challenged, pressure is such that this may be worthy of further debate. The separatist nature of the current workforce does not necessarily relate well to the multi-skilled, multidisciplinary needs of

---

[48] Department of Health (1998) *A First Class Service: Quality in the new NHS* London DoH

[49] Vaughan B, Steiner A, Hanford L (1999) *The Shape of the Team* London King's Fund

practitioners working in Intermediate Care and a review would be timely.

Whole Systems – It has been suggested that, at this point in time, there is insufficient organisational maturity to carry forward major changes to accommodate alternative models of service delivery which will impact on all corners of service provision. Primary Care Groups are in their infancy and are still learning how their patterns of working may impact on whole systems. However, a case can be made that the time has never been more right for radical change since the pressures in the current system have never been greater. Knowledge is being gained of the value of whole systems approaches, using large scale events to identify and work on issues of common concern; exploring and developing what is already working well directly with those concerned and; developing local solutions to local problems to which all the stakeholders are committed. Despite the time and expertise taken to manage these methods well they are gaining credence for their effectiveness at both a strategic and an operational level.

Services to Complement or Substitute – The majority of the projects described within this report have been established with the use of short term, opportunistic funding and have not, as yet impinged on the shifting of money or other resources from one section of the organisation to another. Hence, in this relatively safe way, their introduction has not yet led to a reduction in services elsewhere. Rather they have been seen as a valuable problem solving way of reducing pressure on acute beds, reducing emergency admissions, and keeping children and older people nearer home. However, as the size of Intermediate Care grows, so the impact on other aspects of care will shift. It has been suggested that thinking of the extent of Intermediate Care in terms of the equivalent ward size is a useful way of conceptualising the knock on effects. Thus as the number of patients treated and the number of bed days saved go up it is possible to see how the need for traditional inpatient beds may decrease. This, coupled with an increase in the use of ambulatory services, will inevitably have consequences for the size and shape of acute care services which, in turn, will have a significant impact on both the shape of the workforce and the way in which it works.

In addition the growing recognition that the quality of highly specialised care cannot be sustained unless sufficient numbers of patients are treated at any one single site will also have its influence. Thus it can be argued that the reality of the future will require centralisation of highly specialised tertiary services, development of a range of ambulatory services as technological developments impact on care, a supportive range of intermediate care services and an overall reduction in the size of the secondary care sector.

Conclusion

That there will be changes in future patterns of health care is inevitable and there are already many excellent examples where new models of service delivery are being explored. It is timely to examine just what is happening at both a strategic and an operational level, to open up the debate about options, and to consider the wider implications of these changes.

The development of Intermediate Care cannot be seen in isolation but must be placed in the wider arena, with consideration given to the impact that change in one part of the system will have on the whole organisation, the people who work within it and those who use it. Some thoughts have been set out above as points for debate. No certain answers are offered but questions raised, sometimes around issues which are uncomfortable or difficult to address. It is hoped that they will provide a useful starting point from which others can continue to consider creative new ways of working which are sensitive to patient need.

Part Five

A directory of developments

The primary purpose of this section of the report is to facilitate networking among those people who are interested in developing Intermediate Care services. A brief outline of more than seventy examples has been included, based on details provided by those responsible for offering the service. While information was received from many more sites, the number of entries has been limited by space. Those included reflect the range and type of services being developed in order to offer a snapshot overview of developments. We also anticipate that readers will add information about other schemes which come to their attention over time.

Information has been included about the type and purpose of the service, funding arrangements and, where appropriate, multi-agency involvement. A summary profile of both the patients using the service and the team offering care has been included, as has an indication of the nature and extent of the service. A note of any evaluation being undertaken is also available. In some entries details are either not available or not pertinent to all categories, in which case no entry has been made against that item. Contact details are available in order that links can be made between people with similar interests or those who wish to explore and share ideas and experiences.

The entries have been collated under ten different groupings (see table of contents), some of which are clear cut, such as the nurse-led in-patient services, while for others there is a degree of overlap.

The entries in the directory offer an overview of the activities which were being undertaken at the time that the information was collected. As this is an area of such rapid growth, many of the schemes will already have developed further or may, for one reason or another, have changed form or been discontinued. Understanding why such changes have occurred will, in itself, be of value and offer an opportunity to gain insight into some of the driving or inhibiting forces in introducing new services of this nature.

Finally we would like to publicly thank all the people who so willingly gave us information about their services, whether or not they have been included here. Without their support it would not have been possible to prepare this directory or the accompanying report.

Abbreviations in text

Physiotherapist - physio, PT
Occupational therapist - OT
Speech and language therapist - SaLT
Social worker - SW
Health care assistant/worker - HCA/W
Administrative and clerical staff - A&C
Social services - SS
Residential and Nursing homes - R and N homes

Early discharge

NAME OF NHS TRUST	NORTH MERSEY COMMUNITY (NHS) TRUST	SCUNTHORPE COMMUNITY NHS TRUST. SCUNTHORPE & GOOLE HOSPITALS' TRUST (ACUTE)
NAME OF PROJECT/SCHEME	Rehabilitation at Home Service (Orthopaedics)	The Challenge Fund Scheme
PURPOSE OF SCHEME	To facilitate early discharge of orthopaedic patients requiring both physiotherapy and occupational therapy. To provide quality rehabilitation tailored to clients' home	To facilitate early discharge from hospital thus alleviating the blockage of acute hospital beds. Focus on medically fit patients who can not yet function at home.
MULTI-AGENCY INVOLVEMENT	District nursing service is linked in with the service for patient wound care and anti-coagulant therapy	Social services, the independent sector (nursing home), GPs, 2 Trusts, Sheffield Hallam University.
START DATE	February 1995	January/February 1998.
FUNDING	Recurrent funding from Sefton HA £109,000. Additional £30,000 for Sept. 98 - March 99 from Liverpool HA	Funded through Challenge Fund monies for 1 year. 3 month extension funded locally to complete evaluation.
REASON FOR INTRODUCTION	To facilitate safe and early discharge of orthopaedic patients. Had heard of orthopaedic rehabilitation scheme run in Peterborough and wanted to set up similar model	To develop community based resources for people who were medically fit to be discharged from hospital without losing the opportunity for continued rehabilitation.
LEAD CLINICIAN	Physiotherapist/Co-ordinator	Therapist-led.
LOCATION	In patients' homes.	Nursing home and a residential home.
AVAILABILITY OF SERVICE	8.30-16.30 (8 hours), 7 days a week	Beds - 24 hours. Therapists - Monday-Friday.
ACCESS TO THE SERVICE	Via central telephone point. Team based in local health centre - identifies suitable patients by regularly visiting wards. Referrals from consultants, nurses, therapists	Patients are identified through therapy staff at hospital according to a set of criteria.
CARE OFFERED	Physiotherapy and occupational therapy-based rehabilitation.	The therapists monitor and revise therapy programmes for patients. Home staff implement these programmes and feedback to the therapists. Emphasis on supporting people to regain skill/confidence for independence.
TIME LIMITATION	Patients discharged approx. 6.5 days post-surgery with average 6.5 days home rehabilitation	Average stay is 4-6 weeks.
RESPONSIBILITY FOR DISCHARGE	Physiotherapist/service co-ordinator or OT	Therapists take the lead in consultation with team.
NO. USING SERVICE	4 to 6	6 people can be managed on the scheme.
NO. OVER PREVIOUS MONTH	13	January - December 1998, 36 people on scheme.
AGE RANGE	No age limit. 30-90 year olds have received service	Nursing Home Jan - Dec 1998 - 59-83 years (av 73 yrs). Residential Home 63 - 93 years (av 80 yrs).
TEAM MEMBERS	Physiotherapist x 1.0; occupational therapist x 1.0; 3 support workers (guaranteed 20 hours/week - flex up to 37 hours/week if required); clerical/administration x 0.5.	1.0 x Occupational Therapist and 1.0 x Physiotherapist at Senior I grade. (Other team members are the staff at the two Homes).
MEASURED BY/EVALUATION	Formal evaluation carried out by Edge Hill University College Ormskirk – completed in August 1996. The service has devised its own outcome measures.	Scheme being evaluated by Sheffield Hallam University. The evaluation will include quantitative analysis based on two nationally recognised outcome measure scales and qualitative evaluation based on patient/staff feedback.
IMPACT/OUTCOMES	"... the quality of the individualised rehabilitation experienced by clients in their own homes is such that faster progress towards an optimum health status is achieved up to six weeks after their operation for hip surgery, than if they had received routine care."	
LESSONS LEARNT/PLANS	Thorough planning and extensive communication needed. Initial client group small (max. 3 patients at any one time) in order to monitor progress and safety of the service.	
DOCUMENTATION AVAILABLE	Executive summary of the evaluation. Patient satisfaction questionnaire.	A draft interim report (December 1998) and full report due Spring 1999.
CONTACT	Jenny Kershaw, Physiotherapist/Service Co-ordinator, Rehabilitation at Home Service, Netherton Health Centre, Magdalen Square, Netherton, Liverpool L30 5SP Tel: 0151-524 3840 & 0151-523 5455	Karen Fanthorpe, GM Disability Services, Scunthorpe Community Health Care NHS Trust, Brumby Hospital, East Common Lane, Scunthorpe, North Lincolnshire DN16 1QQ Tel: 01724 29007 Fax: 01724 271016

Early discharge

NAME OF NHS TRUST	OXFORD RADCLIFFE NHS TRUST	BEDFORDSHIRE AND LUTON COMMUNITY NHS TRUST
NAME OF PROJECT/SCHEME	The Home From Hospital Service	Neurological Team (Multi-Disciplinary)
PURPOSE OF SCHEME	To help patients who no longer require hospital care and who may not be eligible for social services support, but remain vulnerable when discharged home.	To facilitate early discharge by providing intensive rehabilitation. To provide rehabilitation at home thereby preventing unnecessary hospital/nursing home admission
MULTI-AGENCY INVOLVEMENT	Scheme developed and run by British Red Cross Society, Social Services, Intensive carer service (funded by HA)	Social Services, District Nursing, Luton & Dunstable Hospital
START DATE	John Radcliffe Hospital – October 1997; extended to Horton Hospital – April 1998	Jan 1994
FUNDING	Funding has been through a Red Cross legacy and the new Winter Health Fund	Bedfordshire HA: £129,276 per annum
REASON FOR INTRODUCTION	To reduce pressure on beds and ensure safer discharge. Key objective of the service was to ensure that people do not remain in hospital any longer than they need, once medical and nursing requirements have been fulfilled.	High level of hospital admission following stroke. "Revolving Door Syndrome". Substantial pressure on continuing care services including long LoS in nursing/ residential homes. High costs associated with home care.
LEAD CLINICIAN	Scheme's co-ordinator	Physiotherapist
LOCATION	At home	In patients' homes and residential homes
AVAILABILITY OF SERVICE	Referrals to co-ordinator 10.00 to 14.00 Mon-Friday	9.00 - 17.00, 7 days a week.
ACCESS TO THE SERVICE	The service is accessed through the co-ordinator in each hospital. Negotiated by volunteer and patient	Referrals to Neurological Team accepted from consultants, PCT, social services, rehab units.
CARE OFFERED	Preparing the home for the patients arrival and meeting them. Transport from hospital. Shopping. Help with meals. Help with mobility. Collection of prescriptions. Relief for carers. Light housework. Emotional support and comfort	Initial assessments, multi-disciplinary assessment, rehabilitation programmes and review.
TIME LIMITATION	Four week period post discharge	Normally 6 months. Time will be extended if appropriate.
RESPONSIBILITY FOR DISCHARGE	Flexible agreement between volunteer worker & family	Therapists
NO. USING SERVICE	Approx 25	50-55
NO. OVER PREVIOUS MONTH	35 referrals with 25 visits	60
AGE RANGE	34-90 years	16-92 years
TEAM MEMBERS	John Radcliffe Site – 3 paid workers, 2 Co-ordinators (20 and 18 hours respectively) and 1 clerical support member (works 12 hours) – these support a team of 13 volunteers that work a variety of flexible hours. Horton Site – 2 Co-ordinators (20 &10 hrs) - support team of volunteers	Superintendent III Physiotherapist x 1; Senior I Physiotherapist x 2; Senior I Occupational Therapist x 2 Rehabilitation Assistants x 3.5.
MEASURED BY/EVALUATION	Collation of statistics. Monitoring forms which collect quantitative and qualitative information	Patient satisfaction audit. Audit of variance from integrated care pathway. Goal achievement.
IMPACT/OUTCOMES	To date no negative evaluations. Ensures a better quality of discharge. An extended service is needed. Difficult to quantify the amount of savings made to the hospital in terms of bed occupancy, and earlier discharges	Team initially involved in stroke rehabilitation. Further funding has meant that the team has expanded and will see patients with progressive neurological conditions. Planning of discharges is more integrated. Team now has a liaison post within the acute unit.
LESSONS LEARNT/PLANS	Need to ensure all clinical areas are aware of service. Aim to expand the service to the A&E department.	Importance of collaboration/communication and robust evaluation methods. Need for interface meetings with acute unit. Expanded roles in the community. Accreditation of cross-skilling.
DOCUMENTATION AVAILABLE		Admission protocol. Integrated care pathway. Patient Information Leaflet.
CONTACT	Renee Robson, Co-ordinator, Oxford Radcliffe NHS Trust, Headington, Oxford OX3 9DU Tel: 01865 221742	Karen Seikus, Team Leader, Neurological team, Disability Resource Centre. Poynters House, Poynters Road, Dunstable, Beds. LU5 4TY. Tel: 01582 709 021

Early discharge

NAME OF NHS TRUST	WAKEFIELD & PONTEFRACT COMMUNITY HEALTH NHS TRUST. COMMUNITY & MENTAL HEALTH	SURREY HAMPSHIRE BORDERS COMMUNITY & MENTAL HEALTH NHS TRUST
NAME OF PROJECT/SCHEME	Immediate Support at Home	Haslemere Intermediate Care Scheme
PURPOSE OF SCHEME	A scheme to facilitate hospital discharge (phase 1) and to prevent hospital/residential care admission (phase 2).	Facilitate discharge or offer an alternative to hospital admission
MULTI-AGENCY INVOLVEMENT	GP, Acute Trust, Social Services	Community Trust. Social Services. Primary Health Care Teams
START DATE	Phase 1 – December 1998. Phase 2 – February 1999	October 1998. Funding has run out - 1 April 1999. Proposal to restart scheme is under consideration
FUNDING	From winter pressures funding. £168,000 (to be shared with the LA with whom the scheme is delivered)	Social Services, Surrey. £20,000
REASON FOR INTRODUCTION	To support waiting list initiative. To provide data to determine the requirement for a 24 hour responsive community nursing service and to offer individuals more choice regarding the location of their care	Small scheme operated with Winter Pressures money 1997/98. Very successful and requested by GPs District Nurses co-ordinate the care for their patients within their existing role.
LOCATION	At home	At home
AVAILABILITY OF SERVICE	24 hours, 7 days a week	8.00 to 21.00, 7 days a week
ACCESS TO THE SERVICE	Phase 1 by the hospital social work team and the community care nurse advisors (district nurse). Phase 2 by the GP Oncall Service, A&E Department and the Emergency Duty Team Social Services	Referrals from GP, district nurse, Case Manager to Clinical Service Manager
CARE OFFERED	A combination of skilled district nursing care and health and social care delivered by unqualified health care support workers and community carers	Personal care; social care
TIME LIMITATION	Phase 1 – max. 28 days. Phase 2 – up to 72 hours.	2-6 weeks
RESPONSIBILITY FOR DISCHARGE	Phase 1 – the Co-ordinators. Phase 2 – the Community Care Advisors (DNs)	District nurse in consultation with the client's GP
NO. USING SERVICE	10-15 Phase 1, 2-3 Phase 2	4
NO. OVER PREVIOUS MONTH	48 Phase 1	4
AGE RANGE	55-95	
TEAM MEMBERS	Phase 1: 1x F grade Co-ordinator. Pool health care support workers employed on an ad hoc basis 'as and when required' plus dedicated community carers. Phase 2: 1.5 x G grade district nurses, 2.5 x B grade health care support workers. These can be supplement enhanced by additional workers from the casual register (all grades)	Support workers grade B x 1.5
MEASURED BY/EVALUATION	Being evaluated within the Trust by the quality evaluation department. Number of referrals. Source of referrals. Length of care. Outcome, patients etc.	Bed days saved. Client independence
IMPACT/OUTCOMES	Number of bed days saved. Number of patients prevented from being admitted to hospital	Not yet completed
LESSONS LEARNT/PLANS	The complexity of working with the local authority whose culture is very different from our own. The need to develop truly integrated budgets to requirement. It is hoped that the local authority and the health authority will continue the scheme.	Effective co-ordination of service is time-consuming. For the scheme to be cost effective and expand, there would need to be time costed to managing the service.
DOCUMENTATION AVAILABLE	Protocols	
CONTACT	Janette Firth, Wakefield & Pontefract Community Health NHS Trust, Featherstone Health Centre, Victoria Street, Featherstone, West Yorkshire, WF7 5EZ	Anne Langhorn, Project Leader – Intermediate Care, Directorate of Clinical Practice Farnham Hospital, Hale Road, Farnham, Surrey GU9 9QL Tel: 01483 782139 Fax: 01483 782217

Early discharge

CAMDEN AND ISLINGTON COMMUNITY HEALTH NHS TRUST	*NAME OF NHS TRUST*
Intermediate Community Based Rehabilitation with Community Rehabilitation Team (CRT)	*NAME OF PROJECT/SCHEME*
To fund generic therapy support workers in the CRT. To enable the Team to provide intermediate community rehabilitation for patients referred from the Whittington Supported Discharge Service and patients with neurological conditions from acute hospitals	*PURPOSE OF SCHEME*
Community Trust. Whittington Hospital Trust. UCL Hospital Trust	*MULTI-AGENCY INVOLVEMENT*
November 1998	*START DATE*
Whole systems funding to run for six months. £30,000 funding until May. Trust will then asses various intermediate care schemes offered	*FUNDING*
To support acute units in providing smoother discharge home and release of hospital bed days	*REASON FOR INTRODUCTION*
Team Leader. Day to day management of service	*LEAD CLINICIAN*
Care is provided in patients' homes in the main - patients may attend Peckwater Centre for physiotherapy	*LOCATION*
9.00 - 17.00 Monday to Friday	*AVAILABILITY OF SERVICE*
Written/telephone referrals according to Service Care Pathway	*ACCESS TO THE SERVICE*
Joint goal setting with Hospital Therapy Service. Home/ Centre based treatment pack. Discharge with appropriate care plan/service in place.	*CARE OFFERED*
No information	*TIME LIMITATION*
CRT will advise hospital of discharge	*RESPONSIBILITY FOR DISCHARGE*
6	*NO. USING SERVICE*
6	*NO. OVER PREVIOUS MONTH*
Mid-age range	*AGE RANGE*
2 rehab assistants employed on OT Technical Instructor grades III to support CRT therapists	*TEAM MEMBERS*
Half-way report and six month evaluation of service	*MEASURED BY/EVALUATION*
Numbers low (given three months operational) to date. Numbers of bed days saved to be assessed	*IMPACT/OUTCOMES*
Difficulties with short term funding. In future would aim to take patients from Supported Discharge Team. Recurring funding required	*LESSONS LEARNT/PLANS*
Care Pathway. Scheme will be written up later in the year	*DOCUMENTATION AVAILABLE*
Dr Steven Luttrell, Team Leader CRT, Peckwater Centre, 6 Peckwater Street, London NW5 2TX Tel: 0171-530 6400	*CONTACT*

Early discharge and admission prevention

COMMUNITY HEALTH SOUTH LONDON NHS TRUST	NAME OF NHS TRUST	OXFORD COMMUNITY NHS TRUST
Rapid Response Team	NAME OF PROJECT/SCHEME	Oxford & Banbury Intensive Community Support Service.
To meet rehabilitation need in own home and prevent hospital admission	PURPOSE OF SCHEME	Prevent admission and facilitate early discharge.
Social services, voluntary services	MULTI-AGENCY INVOLVEMENT	Ocupational therapy. District nursing. Physio. GP. Social services home care (incl. carers and care co-ordinator).
September 1998	START DATE	January 1998
Guy's and St. Thomas Trustees and Health Authority reinvestment. (Funding for three years.)	FUNDING	Winter pressures initially, now whole system money – not yet recurrent.
To prevent long stay in A &E departments and admission to hospital beds.	REASON FOR INTRODUCTION	Ease winter pressure on acute sector.
	LEAD CLINICIAN	District nurse/ occupational therapist
At home	LOCATION	At home
8.30 to 18.00, 7 days a week	AVAILABILITY OF SERVICE	Hours: 8.30 to 16.00, Mon to Fri (to refer) Service daily 7.00 to 22.00 with ability to contact night care if required.
From A & E department to Team Leader on call	ACCESS TO THE SERVICE	Bleeping the co-ordinating nurse or therapist.
Personal care and rehabilitation programme	CARE OFFERED	Social Service care is bought on a block contract. Patients can have up to 8 'units' a day incl night visits. Physio and OT. Nursing from existing team.
6 weeks	TIME LIMITATION	6 weeks
Multi-disciplinary team	RESPONSIBILITY FOR DISCHARGE	The Nurse Co-ordinator and sometimes the therapists.
24 on caseload (approx.)	NO. USING SERVICE	Approx 14-18
26 referrals Jan. 1999	NO. OVER PREVIOUS MONTH	New referrals taken on to scheme approx 16
60 - 85+	AGE RANGE	18-96
1x F grade senior nurse; 3x E grade team leaders;9x rehab support workers;1x Snr I community physio; 1x Snr II OT; 0.5 A&C 3	TEAM MEMBERS	G grade district nurse 0.5 x2, Senior II cccupational therapist x 0.5; care co-ordinatorx 0.5; carers 8 full time; physiotherapist x 0.2.
Randomised control trial commencing April 1999. Activity monitoring.	MEASURED BY/EVALUATION	Activity collated on district nursing service computer data base. Evaluation done by independent freelance social scientist.
Saving hospital bed days	IMPACT/OUTCOMES	Early discharges, admission prevention. Rehabilitation and patients/client either returned to previous function level, or increased function level and/or needs assessed for ongoing care packages.
Activity information	DOCUMENTATION AVAILABLE	Collaborative evaluation – mixture of activity and the free lance reviews. Handout from presentation about the service.
Judith Stagg, Service Manager and Claire Godfrey, Head of Nursing Lambeth Healthcare NHS Trust, 11-13 Rutford Road, London SW16 2DQ Tel: 0818-677 7415 Fax: 0181-664 7012	CONTACT	Karen Kann, Nurse Co-ordinator, Intensive Community Support Service (Oxford) Shotover Centre, Cranford Road, Oxford

Early discharge and admission prevention

SURREY HAMPSHIRE BORDERS COMMUNITY & MENTAL HEALTH NHS TRUST	*NAME OF NHS TRUST*	BEDFORD & SHIRES HEALTH & CARE TRUST (COMMUNITY)
Godalming and Milford Shared Care Scheme	*NAME OF PROJECT/SCHEME*	Intermediate Care Service.
To facilitate early discharge and offer an alternative to hospital admission.	*PURPOSE OF SCHEME*	To facilitate early discharge/reduce inappropriate and unnecessary hospital admissions.
Social Services – hospital and locality. Primary Health Care Team. Community Therapists	*MULTI-AGENCY INVOLVEMENT*	Collaborative working with the acute trust (Bedford Hospital), social services and housing.
September 1998. Pilot extended to March 2000	*START DATE*	April 1997
Surrey Social Services. West Surrey Health Authority (Joint). Originally £30,000 each from SS/HA. SS made extra £20,000 available subsequently	*FUNDING*	From two pilot schemes: Hospital Care at Home and Frail elderly support team. 97/98 £1.5 million in total including hospital. 98/99 £1.55 million, 99/2000 provisionally £1.95 million.
Identified as a need to support primary care services by the Godalming Locality Planning Group.	*REASON FOR INTRODUCTION*	To reduce pressure on beds and help waiting lists.
GP accepts responsibility for patients' care. Referrals from hospital are medically assessed by geriatricians	*LEAD CLINICIAN*	Nurse and therapist – co-ordinators of package of care delivered in the home orcommunity hospitals.
In patients' own homes	*LOCATION*	Care is provided in patients' homes and community hospital.
8.00 to 21.00, 7 days a week	*AVAILABILITY OF SERVICE*	24 hours, 7 days a week
Via GP or Case Manager referral to Co-ordinator or consultant at acute hospital, via Community Liaison nurse	*ACCESS TO THE SERVICE*	District Nurse. GP. Acute Hospitals. Social services. Voluntary sector. Relatives/carers.
Personal care. Social care. Basic nursing care. Physiotherapy and occupational therapy	*CARE OFFERED*	Nursing and therapy care – element of social care if part of rehabilitation programme.
6 weeks	*TIME LIMITATION*	6-8 weeks
Co-ordinator in consultation with client, carer and multidisciplinary team	*RESPONSIBILITY FOR DISCHARGE*	Therapists and nurses
10	*NO. USING SERVICE*	54 maximum
10	*NO. OVER PREVIOUS MONTH*	31
70-94	*AGE RANGE*	Predominantly 70+
Co-ordinator grade G x 0.68; Admin ANC 3 x 0.34; Support Workers grade B x 2 ; Physiotherapist Sen I x 0.26; Occupational Therapist Sen I x 0.26	*TEAM MEMBERS*	Community Team: G grade x4, F grade Rehab Nurse x 0.63, Senior I OT x1 TE, Senior II OT x1, E grades (also covers night service) x6, B grades x9, A grades 3.5, Admin x3 (3) and x 0.5 (2).
Community Trust will produce an evaluation of the first 6 months of the scheme in March 1999	*MEASURED BY/EVALUATION*	Customer satisfaction surveys x2. Currently undertaking clinical audit of Intermediate Care Services.
Not yet identified	*IMPACT/OUTCOMES*	Very few re-admissions (15% between November 1998 and January 1999). Improved communication. Equity of services across North and Mid Bedfordshire. Reduction in bed days at acute hospitals.
	LESSONS LEARNT/PLANS	Increase collaborative working with all agencies – joint bids for funding schemes and new initiatives.
Client records. Client satisfaction survey. Therapy discharge reports. Scheme is currently being written up	*DOCUMENTATION AVAILABLE*	Summary of the scheme.
Anne Langhorn, Project Leader – Intermediate Care, Directorate of Clinical Practice Farnham Hospital, Hale Road, Farnham, Surrey GU9 9QL Tel: 01483 782139 Fax: 01483 782217	*CONTACT*	Noreen Last, Intermediate Care Manager, Shires House, 2nd Floor, 3 Kimbolton Road,Bedford MK40 2NU Tel: 01234 310150 Fax: 01234 310149

Early discharge and admission prevention

SOUTH LONDON COMMUNITY HEALTH NHS TRUST	NAME OF NHS TRUST	SOUTH TEES COMMUNITY AND MENTAL HEALTH NHS TRUST, SOUTH TEES ACUTE HOSPITALS NHS TRUST, STROKE ASSOCIATION, TEES HEALTH, MIDDLESBROUGH SOCIAL SERVICES DEPARTMENT
Rapid Response Team/Supported Discharge	NAME OF PROJECT/SCHEME	Middlesbrough Mobile Rehabilitation Resource Team
RRT – to divert patients who are clinically stable and provide range of care at home. Supported Discharge – to facilitate earlier discharge for those patients who could complete recovery at home	PURPOSE OF SCHEME	To facilitate early discharge and prevent hospital admission
3 Acute Trusts. Community Trust, Southwark and Lewisham Social Services	MULTI-AGENCY INVOLVEMENT	2 hospital trusts as above, Middlesbrough Home Care, Stroke Association.
RRT Winter 1998. SD Winter 1999	START DATE	December 1997
Winter Pressures/waiting list funding	FUNDING	Joint – Tees Health and Middlesbrough Social Services
To maximise use of acute beds but to try and care for older people at home as far as possible.	REASON FOR INTRODUCTION	To provide more care in community settings. Scheme aimed at older people and stroke patients. Recognised how difficult it can be for elderly patients to adjust back into community after a protracted stay in hospital
Geriatricians	LEAD CLINICIAN	Physiotherapist on the team and team leader
A&E. Wards. Day hospital. Patients' homes	LOCATION	In patient's own home
9.00 -20.00, 5 days a week	AVAILABILITY OF SERVICE	Normal working hours – but can be varied if needed. Some cover at weekends and bank holidays
Via nurse co-ordinators	ACCESS TO THE SERVICE	Through GP or consultant referral
Nursing, therapy, social care	CARE OFFERED	Physiotherapy, occupational therapy, home care, family support (strokes)
Approx 6 weeks but some flexibility	TIME LIMITATION	6 weeks
Multi-disciplinary team when patient referred at day hospital	RESPONSIBILITY FOR DISCHARGE	Physio and/or OT
Variable	NO. USING SERVICE	20
Variable	NO. OVER PREVIOUS MONTH	20 (Jan 1999)
Mean age 81. No fixed age but majority 65+, have occasionally taken younger people	AGE RANGE	Strokes – any age; others 65+
Approx: 3 x G/F Co-ordinators, Rehab Support Workers, F grade Nurses x 3, Acute contribution OT/Physio x 3. SW's x 2, B grade x 8, Consultant Geriatrician and specialist Registrars also involved	TEAM MEMBERS	Supt III physiotherapist x 1;Senior occupational therapist x 1; rehabilitation assistants x 1.07; clerical support x 0.32;family support E x 1.07; secretarial support x 0.37
By agency. Collective inter agency. By external evaluation of various elements	MEASURED BY/EVALUATION	Patient/Carer questionnaires. Evaluation to be done by University of Teeside. Modified Barthel Index
Small numbers but collective impact across the area significant. Diverts people from long term care. More appropriate to try and rehab people in their own homes	IMPACT/OUTCOMES	Too soon to say
Lead in time always longer than you anticipate. Stop/start funding and uncertainty has an impact. Recruiting the right calibre of worker for rehab support worker is critical	LESSONS LEARNT/PLANS	Need much closer links with acute hospital therapists. Need involvement of SaLT. To roll service out to the rest of the District, funding needs to be available. Rehabilitation and recovery service to complement this team.
Operational policies	DOCUMENTATION AVAILABLE	
Barbara Hills, Locality Manager Tel: 0171-771 3914 Sally Brooks, Locality Manager Tel: 0171-771 5832	CONTACT	Mrs Gail McCraike, Team Leader, The Lodge, Wenthome Hospital, Acklam Road, Middlesbrough, TS5 4EE Tel: 01642 813144 x313 Fax: 01642 822717

Admission prevention

COMMUNITY HEALTH SOUTH LONDON NHS TRUST	NAME OF NHS TRUST	CHESTER AND HALTON COMMUNITY NHS TRUST
Rapid Response Team	NAME OF PROJECT/SCHEME	Hawthornes (intermediate care)
To meet rehabilitation need in own home and prevent hospital admission	PURPOSE OF SCHEME	To facilitate early discharge. To provide extensive rehabilitation. Increasingly to revent admisison to hospital.
Social services, voluntary services.	MULTI-AGENCY INVOLVEMENT	Community, hospital, social services.
September 1998. (Funding for three years.)	START DATE	January 1997
Guy's and St. Thomas Trustees and Health Authority reinvestment	FUNDING	Provided by Health Authority through winter pressures monies - £58,000 annually.
To prevent long stay in A &E departments and inappropriate admission to hospital beds	REASON FOR INTRODUCTION	Gap in services in the community for helping patients to go back to home circumstances.
	LEAD CLINICIAN	Led by nursing/paramedical staff and social service panel. Work supported by care assistants, psychologist.
At home	LOCATION	Social Service residential home
8.30 to 18.00, 7 days a week.	AVAILABILITY OF SERVICE	24 hours, 7 days a week.
From A & E department to Team Leader on call	ACCESS TO THE SERVICE	Any professional (hospital, GP, social services) can refer to a multi disciplinary panel which meets reguarly to assess patients's suitabiity for rehabiitation.
Personal care and rehabilitation programme	CARE OFFERED	Extensive rehabilitation.
6 weeks	TIME LIMITATION	Up to 6 weeks.
Multidisciplinary team	RESPONSIBILITY FOR DISCHARGE	Multi disciplinary team review and patient/carer.
24 on caseload (approximately)	NO. USING SERVICE	July 1998-Jan 1999. 26 Admissions, 26 discharges.
26 referrals in month of Jan. 1999	NO. OVER PREVIOUS MONTH	
2 x 60-65, 5 x 65-74, 12 x 75-84, 7 x 85+	AGE RANGE	55 - 80+
1x F grade senior nurse; 3x E grade team leaders; 9x B rehabilitation support workers; 1x Snr I community physiotherapist; 1x Snr II occupational therapist; 0.5 A&C 3	TEAM MEMBERS	Physiotherapist x 0.5; occupational therapist x 0.5; district nurse x 0.4; care assistants x 1.5 plus existing home care assistant; psychologist x 01 hours per week.
Randomised control trial commencing April 1999. Activity monitoring	MEASURED BY/EVALUATION	Internal audits. Admission, discharge, follow up at 3 months.
Saving hospital bed days	IMPACT/OUTCOMES	Patients returned home. Patient satisfaction. Bed blockage in acute hospital stopped.
	LESSONS LEARNT/PLANS	Took time to market. Now full capacity. Needs to have mainstream funding.
Activity information	DOCUMENTATION AVAILABLE	System of continuing internal audit produces quarterly reports monitoring use of service.
Judith Stagg, Service Manager & Claire Godfrey, Head of Nursing Lambeth Healthcare NHS Trust, 11-13 Rutford Road, London SW16 2DQ Tel: 0818-677 7415 Fax: 0181-664 7012	CONTACT	Mrs Malkia Ibbotson, Primary Care Facilitator, North Cheshire Health, Lister Road,Runcorn Tel: 01928 593000 Fax: 01928 569432

Admission prevention

AYLESBURY VALE HEALTHCARE – COMMUNITY TRUST	*NAME OF NHS TRUST*	MILTON KEYNES GENERAL NHS HOSPITAL TRUST
Weston Project	*NAME OF PROJECT/SCHEME*	GP in A & E (Primary Care Pilot Project).
To prevent hospital/nursing home/residential home admission and to assist with early discharge. The project is open to all adults.	*PURPOSE OF SCHEME*	Appropriate use of A&E and Primary Care services by the assessment/triage of patients self referring to A&E. Improve patient throughput. Educate patients about appropriate health care provision. Improve links between hospital and community.
Working collaboratively with social service (accredited as a social care provider by Bucks, awaiting accreditation with Herts), community physiotherapy and OT.	*MULTI-AGENCY INVOLVEMENT*	Community Trust (District Nursing). Social services. GP practices. Health information. NHD Direct.
May 1998	*START DATE*	October 1998.
Winter Pressure money plus money from Region (land sales from Community Trust). £450,000 - 2 years	*FUNDING*	Whole Systems funding, 'Winter Pressures' - £70,000.
To help with managing winter pressures. To develop a model for intermediate care using a whole systems approach	*REASON FOR INTRODUCTION*	Pressure on beds.
A GP is Chair of the Project Board - responsible for project direction and for overseeing management team.	*LEAD CLINICIAN*	GP leads assessment and triage process.
People's homes.	*LOCATION*	A&E Dept. Milton Keynes General Hospital.
Care available from 8.00 to 22.30, plus 4 nights, 7 days a week including Bank Holidays. Referral access to the project is currently Mon-Sun from 8.30 to 17.00. Night time referrals possible from April.	*AVAILABILITY OF SERVICE*	11.00 to 19.00, Monday to Friday
Referral can be made by GP, district nurse, physiotherapist, occupational therapist, social services, hospital.	*ACCESS TO THE SERVICE*	Direct access by patients self presenting in A&E.
Assessed by one of a team of district nurses. Between one and five visits per day. Visits are also made by the Co-ordinator to the clients home. At all times the patient remains under the clinical responsibility of their own GP.	*CARE OFFERED*	Expert medical opinion. Health education. District nursing assessment.
Average length of stay - 12 days. Patients are on project from 1-30 days, though 2 weeks is the usual maximum	*TIME LIMITATION*	Not applicable
Co-ordinator liaises with the client, district nurse and Social service to agree an end date.	*RESPONSIBILITY FOR DISCHARGE*	Lead GP
12 (dependent on level of dependency)	*NO. USING SERVICE*	14 per day
25	*NO. OVER PREVIOUS MONTH*	280
Over 16 (most are 75+)	*AGE RANGE*	All
Project leader x .60 Trust grade 11; nurse co-ordinator x 1.00 Trust grade 11; health care support workers x 9.56 Trust grade B; volunteers x 3. OT and physio as needed.	*TEAM MEMBERS*	GP x 1. G grade Community Nurse x 1.
Public Health Resource Unit, Headington, Oxford. London Health Economics Consortium. Audit tool to be developed.	*MEASURED BY/EVALUATION*	Patient & staff satisfaction questionnaires.
Improved communications between health and social services. Prevention of hospital admission in approximately half of the total number (120) referrals. Fast tracking for SS assessments, physio & OT.	*IMPACT/OUTCOMES*	Anticipated improvements in utilisation of A&E services; increase more appropriate use of NHS direct, Health information. Changes in public perception.
Role out the project to the PCG. Expand the service to enable referrals to be taken 24 hours. Facilitate early discharge from medical wards and surgery.	*LESSONS LEARNT/PLANS*	The importance of good preparation.
	DOCUMENTATION AVAILABLE	Project outline – protocol for assessment/triage.
Nicole Cox – Project Leader. Mary Burton – Nurse Co-ordinator, West Project Office, Wendover Health Centre, Aylesbury Road, Wendover HP22 6LD Tel: 01296 621017 Fax: 01296 621019	*CONTACT*	Alison Fenn-Coles, Head of Nursing, Milton Keynes General NHS Trust, Milton Keynes General Hospital, Standing Way, Eaglestone, Milton Keynes MK6 5LD Tel: 01908 660033 bleep 1021

Admission prevention

COMMUNITY HEALTH SHEFFIELD	NAME OF NHS TRUST	BURY & ROCHDALE HEALTH AUTHORITY
Community Rehabilitation Unit (CRU)	NAME OF PROJECT/SCHEME	Bury & Rochdale Rapid Response Service
To provide multidisciplinary rehabilitation to elderly patients in the south of Sheffield.	PURPOSE OF SCHEME	To prevent unnecessary hospital admissions.
Kersal Mount Nursing Home. Community Health Sheffield NHS Trust.	MULTI-AGENCY INVOLVEMENT	Private Sector Nursing Homes. Bury & Rochdale Health Authority. Bury HC Trust. Rochdale HC Trust. Bury Social Services. Rochdale Social Services. Bury & Rochdale Primary Health Care Teams.
November 1996	START DATE	November 1997
Sheffield Health Authority provision for Elderly Rehabilitation following closure of Nether Edge Hospital.	FUNDING	Winter Pressures monies matched with Health Authority funding and GP funds.
Closure of Rehabilitation Hospital therefore reduction in Sheffield of beds for the elderly and a need to look at alternative ways of providing elderly rehabilitation.	REASON FOR INTRODUCTION	To help solve the bed crisis especially during the winter.
Nursing home and outreach.	LOCATION	Patient's home; nursing home.
In-patients: 24 hours, 7 days a week	AVAILABILITY OF SERVICE	24 hours. Referrals 9.00 to 19.00 weekdays; 9.00 to 17.00, weekends and Bank Holidays.
By referral from consultants based at the Royal Hallamshire Hospital .	ACCESS TO THE SERVICE	By any GP signed up to the scheme or by the hospital discharge Co-ordinators.
Rehabilitation to elderly patients – physio, OT, SaLT, dietician, nursing and medical.	CARE OFFERED	24 hour nursing care either in a patient's home – Rapid Home Support (RHS), or nursing home care – Intermediate Managed Care (IMC).
20 weeks	TIME LIMITATION	RHS = 3/4 days. IMC = maximum of 14 days.
Joint between consultant and therapist. All discharges are planned and agreed with outreach in patient's home.	RESPONSIBILITY FOR DISCHARGE	Rapid Response Team sister in conjunction with the patients GP.
20 inpatients and 5 patients on out reach.	NO. USING SERVICE	
Jan 1999 = 17 new patients.	NO. OVER PREVIOUS MONTH	January 1999 = 65 referrals.
72-98	AGE RANGE	Over 65
Team Leader – Job share between physio/OT(0.5 PT x0.5 OT). 2x 1 Senior I physio x 0.5; 1 Senior I OT x 1.0; 1 Senior I occupational therapist x 0.5;. 3 therapy assists x1.0 + 1 therapy assistant x 0.5.Nursing Manager.	TEAM MEMBERS	2 RGN full time G grade. 1 RGN 1/2 time F grade. 20 (variable) Bank support workers B grade. 12 hours clerical support.
Bed nights; Community contacts; Discharge destination; medicine diagnosis.	MEASURED BY/EVALUATION	Monitoring and Evaluation data required was included in the original specification. An interim evaluation of the scheme has also been completed by the Nuffield Institute.
Therapy outcome measures. Elderly Mobility Scores. Barthel.	IMPACT/OUTCOMES	Proven saving of hospital bed days. Contributes to maintaining people for longer in their own homes. Another resource for GPs. Advice to GPs. Helps Nursing Homes keep up to date with acutely ill patients.
The positive aspects of 'half-way home' environment. The positives and negatives of this type of collaboration between the private and public sector.	LESSONS LEARNT/PLANS	Much improved understanding of other agencies which we hope to further develop. Expand the service – especially by involving all GPs so all residents of Bury and Rochdale have equal access.
Annual report 1997. Statistics of Outcome measure/ length of stay etc.	DOCUMENTATION AVAILABLE	Presentation package available – summarises service.
Julie Rees/Anne Bartholomew – Team Leaders, CRU, 115 Manchester Road, Sheffield S10 Tel: 0114- 266 4252 Fax: 0114-266 4325	CONTACT	Gwen Sharpe, Bury & Rochdale Health Authority, 21 Silver Street, Bury BL9 0EN Tel: 0161-762 3112 Response Team, c/o BARDOC, Carne House, Parsons Lane, Bury BL9 0JT Tel: 0161-763 4242 Fax: 0161- 763 4555

Admission prevention

MILTON KEYNES COUNCIL	NAME OF NHS TRUST	SOUTH WEST LONDON TPP
Emergency Response Service	NAME OF PROJECT/SCHEME	Integrated Care Project
The aim of the project was to prove the need for an Emergency Home Care Service to respond to emergency social care needs out of office hours	PURPOSE OF SCHEME	To prevent/reduce emergency admissions to hospital. To facilitate timely discharge. To prevent delayed discharge.
Milton Keynes Neighbourhood Services. Milton Keynes Health	MULTI-AGENCY INVOLVEMENT	
June 1996	START DATE	January 1997
Buckingham Social Services. Health Authority and Milton Keynes Housing. Total of £75,000 over 3 years - joint funding	FUNDING	Pump priming from Challenge Fund, now core.
The aim of the project was to prove the need for an Emergency Home Care Service to respond to emergency social care needs out of office hours.	REASON FOR INTRODUCTION	Rise in emergency admission rate and delayed discharge. Difficulties in admission because of bed shortages.
Service is managed through home care - part of neighbourhood services within Milton Keynes Council.	LEAD CLINICIAN	
In people's homes	LOCATION	Care is provided in the patient's home but community hospital and nursing home placement are arranged where appropriate.
Mon-Fri 17.30 - 9.00, Sat-Sun 21.00 - 9.00 – an out of hours emergency service.	AVAILABILITY OF SERVICE	24 hours, 7 dayas a week.
Calls are made through Housing Alarm Centre, which then calls out carers. Referrals can be made by another professional eg. through A & E, emergency social work team. through Housing Alarm service, through GPs or local community nursing service.	ACCESS TO THE SERVICE	By single points of contact - one for intermediate care, one for discharge planning team. GPs, nurses, social workers, patients, relatives/carers can all refer/self-refer.
Social care by experienced home carers.	CARE OFFERED	In-patient and home based intermediate care identification of 'at risk' patients care planning and case management – Discharge Alert Register.
One off visit – appropriate referrals to other agencies made as needed next working day.	TIME LIMITATION	Length of stay targets for intermediate care. No time limits for Discharge Alert Register (DA).
	RESPONSIBILITY FOR DISCHARGE	Primary nurse.
18	NO. USING SERVICE	IC = 30 per month. DA = 30 per month.
27 - 91 years	NO. OVER PREVIOUS MONTH	1C 30. DA 30
	AGE RANGE	Over 16 years.
Not available	TEAM MEMBERS	Intermediate care is purchased from other providers. Discharge Planning Team – Co-ordinator = SMP 16, Administrator = grade 5, Grade G = 1, Grade F = 2.8.
Detailed data on contacts collected. Patient satisfaction survey carried out	MEASURED BY/EVALUATION	Quarterly report – prevention of admissions, length of stay, supported discharge, readmissions, discharge destination. King's Fund audit.
Benefits for the hospital (A&E). Carer able to be called to take people home and settle them after perhaps a fall.	IMPACT/OUTCOMES	Reduced emergency admission rates.
	LESSONS LEARNT/PLANS	IT strategy – links to A&E depts and social services. Care Pathway for COPD, older person's assessment, falls prevention strategy, risk scoring.
	DOCUMENTATION AVAILABLE	Annual and quarterly reports.
Mary Douglas, Home Care Co-ordinator; Dorothy Croke, Home Care Services Manager, 3 St Giles Mew, Stony Stratford, Milton Keynes MK11 1HT Tel: 01908 265682 Fax: 01908 260634	CONTACT	Heather Maughan, Discharge Planning Co-ordinator, SWLTPP, Discharge Planning Team 157A Cannon Hill Lane, London SW20 9DA Tel: 0181-542 2421 Fax: 0181-542 2123

Community rehabilitation - home based

GLOUCESTERSHIRE HEALTH AUTHORITY; EAST GLOUCESTERSHIRE NHS TRUST; GLOUCESTERSHIRE ROYAL NHS TRUST; GLOUCESTERSHIRE SOCIAL SERVICES DEPARTMENT; SEVERN NHS TRUST	NAME OF NHS TRUST	NOTTINGHAM COMMUNITY HEALTH TRUST
Community Rehabilitation Scheme	NAME OF PROJECT/SCHEME	Community Rehabilitation.
Prevent inappropriate, avoidable admission into institutional care and promote recovery to appropriate level of independence.	PURPOSE OF SCHEME	To facilitate early discharge and avoid admission. Provide community based rehabilitation for people who have had a stroke, and their carers.
Joint initiative between health and social services.	MULTI-AGENCY INVOLVEMENT	Social services, health, voluntary.
3 Pilot schemes – 1st started 1.10.98, 2nd started 1.12.98	START DATE	May 1996
Joint funding – health and social services	FUNDING	Joint finance/health authority, waiting list money.
Managing demand	REASON FOR INTRODUCTION	To reduce pressures on beds. To build up multi-disciplinary team working in community with an emphasis on providing rehabilitation services for the elderly.
Scheme is managed by social services. Three pilot schemes are led by a physiotherapist	LEAD CLINICIAN	In the north, a specialist nurse; in the south, a physiotherapist.
At home	LOCATION	At home
24 hours, 7 days a week	AVAILABILITY OF SERVICE	8.00 to 22.00, 7 days a week.
Single point of contact (tel. no) - specific for each pilot	ACCESS TO THE SERVICE	Referral by phone/fax from multi-disc. hospital staff. Central referral point – medical agreement is needed.
Care appropriate to patients needs to assist in managing crisis – this may be social/personal care or health care.	CARE OFFERED	Nursing, physio/OT, mental health, speech therapy, social work. Co-workers – an auxiliary nurse and a communiuty care assistant combine health and social care provision.
Expected to last a maximum of 6 weeks	TIME LIMITATION	
In consultation between key worker and patient's GP	RESPONSIBILITY FOR DISCHARGE	Keyworker/clinicians.
Variable	NO. USING SERVICE	100
Average 20-30 across pilots	NO. OVER PREVIOUS MONTH	
No age criterion but most are 75 years plus	AGE RANGE	Stroke -16 onwards but mainly elderly. Care programme - 16-65. Intermediate care – 65 onwards.
Grade G district nurse x 0.5; Sn 1 physiotherapist x 1.5; Sn 1 occupational therapist x1.5; domiciliary care assessor x 1; home care support workers x 3; 3 A&C grade 3 x 0.5.	TEAM MEMBERS	There are 40 team members (multi disciplinary) of all types and grades.
Evaluation in place. Interim review due March 1999; full evaluation October 1999	MEASURED BY/EVALUATION	Action research (stroke). Randomised control trial (3 years).
Reduction in inappropriate admissions to hospital (part of evaluation process)	IMPACT/OUTCOMES	Stroke outcome – advice given to health authority to expand service.
	LESSONS LEARNT/PLANS	Different strands to service presently forming into a more cohesive service ie. community rehabilitation, removing all the different titles – as it is confusing.
Service specification and evaluation framework; information leaflets.	DOCUMENTATION AVAILABLE	Leaflets, reports, plans.
Jackie Huck, Gloucestershire Health Authority, Victoria Warehouse, The Docks, Gloucester GL1 2EL Tel: 01452 318827 Fax: 01452 318810	CONTACT	Anita Dixon, Rehab Co-ordinator, Mary Potter Hostel, Gregory Boulevard, Nottingham, NG7 7HY Tel: 0115 9784561

Community rehabilitation - home based

HULL & HOLDERNESS COMMUNITY HEALTH NHS TRUST	*NAME OF NHS TRUST*	**HULL & HOLDERNESS COMM. HEALTH NHS TRUST, EAST YORKSHIRE COMMUNITY HEALTHCARE NHS TRUST, SCUNTHORPE COMMUNITY HEALTH NHS TRUST**
Integrated Intermediate Care Service	*NAME OF PROJECT/SCHEME*	East Riding Intermediate Care Project (ERIC.P)
To avoid as far as possible, inappropriate admissions to hospital, to reduce the lengths of stay in acute hospital settings and improve discharge arrangements by providing a rapid response to hospital wards' request for intervention. To provide an integrated joint health and social services approach to care delivery.	*PURPOSE OF SCHEME*	To offer a therapeutic rehabilitation and recuperation service. To provide direct rapid response. To facilitate early discharge from hospital. To provide on-going multi-agency assessment and treatment. To further improve multi-disciplinary co-ordination to improved discharge arrangements and assist with early discharge.
Health, Social Services (Kingston upon Hull City Council) Age Concern, Stroke Association, Acute hospitals	*MULTI-AGENCY INVOLVEMENT*	Health (all 3 Comm. Trusts, Social Services (East Riding of Yorkshire Council), professions allied to medicine
October 1998	*START DATE*	October 1998
£315k Waiting List Initiative funding (6 months effect); £106k Special Transitional Grant (STG) moneys (6 months effect)	*FUNDING*	£134.5k Waiting List Initiative funding (6 month effect); £162k Special Transitional Grant (STG) monies (6 month effect). (Plus £412k expected budget implications for residential/nursing care beds and priority care teams.)
Success of pilot service 1 Jan 98 to 31 March 98 (Winter Pressures monies). To offer alternative to hospitalisation.	*REASON FOR INTRODUCTION*	To meet Government initiatives for Care in the Community.
District nursing	*LEAD CLINICIAN*	Health Co-ordinator and Assessment Officer (SS)
At patient's home or within identified social services residential resource centre, if more intensive care needed	*LOCATION*	People's homes
24 hours, 7 days a week	*AVAILABILITY OF SERVICE*	Varies from area to area
Directly via the team via one telephone number	*ACCESS TO THE SERVICE*	Via each area team office
Individualised and holistic care.Potential for rehabilitation within person's own home or identified bed within Social Services res. resource centre for more intensive care.	*CARE OFFERED*	Potential for rehabilitation within persons own home or identified bed within Social Services residential resource centre for more intensive care.
6 weeks	*TIME LIMITATION*	6 weeks
The team	*RESPONSIBILITY FOR DISCHARGE*	The team
Approx 40 dependent upon case mix	*NO. USING SERVICE*	Approx 10 in each area dependent upon casemix.
21 Int. Care Service, 43 Evening District Nursing Service.	*NO. OVER PREVIOUS MONTH*	Varies over areas
18 years +	*AGE RANGE*	65 years + with the odd exception
Nurses - 0.43 x I grade (team leader), 0.57 x H grade, 2 x G grades, 1x acting F grade, 2 x acting E grade, 2.85 x D grades; 1.80 support worker (health); 4.40 x care officer (SS); 1x C grade, 1x Senior III OT; 1x Senior III physiotherapist; 1x A&C 3. 2 sessions psychology	*TEAM MEMBERS*	6x Assessment Officers (Social Services) – one per team. In addition each team had District Nursing Health co-ordinators. The staffing levels varied from area to area. PAMs input available in East Yorkshire Comm Trust
Statistical information. Integrated Care Pathways. Barthel index. Joint Care Plans. Subjective measures: Satisfaction Questionnaires (Patient/Carer); Satisfaction Questionnaires (Referring Agent)	*MEASURED BY/EVALUATION*	Statistical information (activity sheets, progress sheets etc.); Referral Pathways; Joint Care Plans. Subjective Measures: Satisfaction Questionnaires (Patient/Carer); Satisfaction Questionnaire (Referring Agent).
Rehab effect is evident, care is consistent, minimal overlap of roles except when necessary which provides an efficient team, individualised/ holistic care to each patient in their own home - encourages motivation and enthusiasm, rapid response to referral, ongoing continuous assessment of patient whilst with ICS. Providing after care services with detailed history enables cost effective service. Family/carers more closely involved with rehab	*IMPACT/OUTCOMES*	Achieved the aims around reducing avoidable admissions and facilitating early discharge. Of those patents using the scheme approximately 50% prevented a hospital admission and 50% were discharged early from hospital.
Evaluation of Initial Pilot. Operational Policy	*DOCUMENTATION AVAILABLE*	Interim Evaluation Reportt. Operational Policy.
Angie Mason, SDM, Hull & Holderness Community Health NHS Trust, Victoria House, Park Street, Hull HU2 8TD Tel: 01482 223191 Fax: 01482 229668	*CONTACT*	Tina Kingdom, Health Co-ordinator, Hull & Holderness Community Health NHS Trust Rosedale, Hedon, Hull

Community rehabilitation - home based

NAME OF NHS TRUST	**SURREY HAMPSHIRE BORDERS COMMUNITY & MENTAL HEALTH NHS TRUST**	**SURREY HAMPSHIRE BORDERS COMMUNITY & MENTAL HEALTH NHS TRUST**
NAME OF PROJECT/SCHEME	Rehabilitation at Home – Surrey Heath	Farnham – Intermediate Care
PURPOSE OF SCHEME	To facilitate early discharge	To facilitate discharge referred in by multidisciplinary team and offer an alternative to hospital admission.
MULTI-AGENCY INVOLVEMENT	Acute hospital – Frimley Park Hospital, St Peters, Chertsey. Social Services. Community Trust PCHTs	Social Services. Community Trust. Primary Health Care Teams. Acute Trusts.
START DATE	September 1995	November 1998
FUNDING	West Surrey Health Authority, about £112,00 per year	West Surrey Health Authority - £69,000 per year.
REASON FOR INTRODUCTION	The Surrey Heath locality has no community hospital - rehabilitation for elderly clients took place alongside acute care. Rehab at home increased options and reduced length of stay.	As part of the review of Farnham and Fleet Community Hospital, the scheme was introduced to enable a reduction in the number of GP beds.
LEAD CLINICIAN	Consultant Physician in Geriatric Medicine	Therapist to set goals and monitor progress. 'Key worker' will change according to each clients needs.
LOCATION	At home	Home based scheme
AVAILABILITY OF SERVICE	8.00 to 21.00, 7 days a week	8.00 to 21.00, 7 days a week.
ACCESS TO THE SERVICE	Community Liaison nurses in acute hospital; patients identified at multidisciplinary team meetings. then confirmed with co-ordinator.	Referral from GP or district nurse to Co-ordinator. Identified at multidisciplinary team meetings in acute and community hospital and referred to Co-ordinator.
CARE OFFERED	Personal care. Social care. Physiotherapy. Occupational therapy. Basic nursing care under direction of the patients' district nurse.	Personal care. Social care. Physiotherapy. Occupational therapy. Basic nursing care under the direction of the clients District Nurse.
TIME LIMITATION	6 weeks	2-6 weeks
RESPONSIBILITY FOR DISCHARGE	The Co-ordinator in consultation with client, carers and multidisciplinary team	Co-ordinator in consultation with client, carer, GP and multidisciplinary team
NO. USING SERVICE	12	8
NO. OVER PREVIOUS MONTH	10	7
AGE RANGE	60-98	65-92
TEAM MEMBERS	Co-ordinator grade G x .65. Physiotherapist Senior I x 0.35. Occupational Therapist Senior I x 0.27 . Multi-disciplinary Health Care Support Workers grade B x 4.00. Administration A&C 3 x 0.53.	Co-ordinator grade G x 0.25; Physiotherapist Senior I x 0.26; Occupational Therapist Senior I x 0.26; Administration ANC 3 x 0.26; Support workers x 2.
MEASURED BY/EVALUATION	Evaluated by University of Surrey in 1997. Barthel scores. Cost. Outcomes for clients	Evaluated by the Community Trust in consultation with GPs and district nurses. Barthel scores.
IMPACT/OUTCOMES	Elderly Care Unit at Frimley Park Hospital did a survey and found a significant reduction in average length of stay. Reduction in size of care packages; if required clients able to remain in their own houses instead of considering residential care	Not yet completed
LESSONS LEARNT/PLANS	To integrate with other schemes, initiatives in the locality. To extend the scheme to accept referrals from PHCT's and Day Hospitals	To be identified after evaluation of first 6 months of the scheme.
DOCUMENTATION AVAILABLE	OT has produced case study write up of 2 stroke patients	Scheme is currently being written up.
CONTACT	Anne Langhorn, Project Leader – Intermediate Care, Directorate of Clinical Practice Farnham Hospital, Hale Road, Farnham, Surrey GU9 9QL Tel: 01483 782139 Fax: 01483 782217	Anne Langhorn, Project Leader – Intermediate Care, Directorate of Clinical Practice Farnham Hospital, Hale Road, Farnham, Surrey GU9 9QL Tel: 01483 782139 Fax: 01483 782217

Community rehabilitation - home based

NAME OF NHS TRUST	MERTON AND SUTTON COMMUNITY NHS TRUST	SURREY HAMPSHIRE BORDERS COMMUNITY & MENTAL HEALTH NHS TRUST
NAME OF PROJECT/SCHEME	Joint Rehabilitation and Assessment Project	Crisis at Home – North East Hampshire
PURPOSE OF SCHEME	To facilitate timely discharge. To prevent unnecessary hospital admission. To facilitate clients with neurological conditions eg. multiple sclerosis to stay in their own home environment longer. By providing specialist nursing therapy, and social care within the home environment	To offer an alternative to hospital admission
MULTI-AGENCY INVOLVEMENT	Jointly commissioned project between London Borough of Sutton Housing, SS Department and HA	Hampshire Social Services
START DATE	July 1996	March 1996
FUNDING	Joint funding – Social Services and Health	North and Mid Hampshire Health Authority
REASON FOR INTRODUCTION	To improve the interface between primary and secondary care.To meet gaps for longer term maintenance and rehabilitation of clients following hospital discharge.To reduce fragmentation of out-reach services. To prevent inappropriate admission to residential and nursing care homes.To reduce hospital admission for people requiring intensive rehabilitation and social care support.	To reduce the number of inappropriate admissions to acute hospital
LEAD CLINICIAN	Senior OT Acting Team Leader	GP – to retain medical responsibility
LOCATION	Home based	At home
AVAILABILITY OF SERVICE	9.00 - 17.00 Monday to Friday	8.00 to 21.00, 7 days a week
ACCESS TO THE SERVICE	Open referral scheme - anyone including patient can make referral, anyone on team can accept referral	Must be an assessment by GP. GP or district nurses identify patients, patient is assessed - referral made to Co-ordinator of scheme. Some referrals come via SS.
CARE OFFERED	Detailed initial assessment (joint health and social services). Assessment by an OT, Physio, SaLT, and Home Care assessor as appropriate. Jointly agreed goals (team, client, carer). Treatment if appropriate to level of package. Advice, support and training for carers	Personal care. Social care. Basic nursing care under the direction of the client's district nurse.
TIME LIMITATION	Majority within 6-8 weeks; more complex cases longer	2 weeks
RESPONSIBILITY FOR DISCHARGE	The team in partnership with client and carers	Co-ordinator in consultation with district nurse.
NO. USING SERVICE	Average 22	6
NO. OVER PREVIOUS MONTH	34 patient treated. 14 assessments	8 (Availability of Winter Pressures funding enable the scheme to increase the availability of episodes of care.)
AGE RANGE	From 17 years	
TEAM MEMBERS	1.25 x Physio, 1.0 x OT, 0.25 x SLT, 0.50 x Therapy Assistant, 0.32 x Specialist Nurse, 0.40 x A&C	Co-ordinator grade G x 0.25 WTE. Support Workers grade B x 2. Administration A&C 3 x 0.20.
MEASURED BY/EVALUATION	Currently being evaluated by external consultants commissioned by Merton and Sutton, Wandsworth HA	Community Trust – bed days saved. Cost. Outcome for client.
IMPACT/OUTCOMES	Outcome measures used, ie. Teler TM, COOP, Personal Problem Identification Rating Scale, demonstrate positive outcome following therapeutic intervention. Surveys show how much clients/carers value service	
LESSONS LEARNT/PLANS	Set up by multi-agency steering group. Team leader taken by a clinician - should have been at higher grade. Exit strategy needed once short-term money finished.	Basic scheme can be enlarged to extend range of services offered, by the inclusion of other disciplines ie. Physiotherapy/occupational therapy. This can then include diversions from A&E and support for early discharge.
DOCUMENTATION AVAILABLE	Referral criteria, service leaflets, yearly reports	
CONTACT	Mrs Donna Bayliss, Acting Team Leader, JRAP, Carshalton War Memorial Hospital, The Park, Carshalton, Surrey SM5 3DB Tel: 0181-669 3621	Anne Langhorn, Project Leader – Intermediate Care, Directorate of Clinical Practice Farnham Hospital, Hale Road, Farnham, Surrey GU9 9QL Tel: 01483 782139 Fax: 01483 782217

Community rehabilitation - home based

MERTON AND SUTTON COMMUNITY NHS TRUST	NAME OF NHS TRUST	BEDFORDSHIRE AND LUTON COMMUNITY TRUST
Community Stroke Rehabilitation Team	NAME OF PROJECT/SCHEME	Elderly Rehabilitation Team
Timely discharge and prevention of unnecessary clinical admissions	PURPOSE OF SCHEME	Facilitate and support early discharge. Support to prevent hospital admission.
Local acute Trusts, Social Service OT's, SWs, care managers, local rehab units, vol. sector eg. Stroke clubs.	MULTI-AGENCY INVOLVEMENT	Social Services, Acute Trust
Community Stroke Team started as a three year project in May 1994. Now funded by HA. Approx. £170,00 pa.	START DATE	July 1996
Funded by Health Authority. Waiting list monies have funded an Enhanced Recovery Project (ERP)for 6 patients. This project is enabling very acute stroke patients to be discharged very early into community for care at home.	FUNDING	Source:Health Authority, Challenge Fund, Winter pressures monies. Total: £249,215. £26,853 (travel, telephone, dressings etc.)
Services were very fragmented; need for a co-ordinated approach	REASON FOR INTRODUCTION	Stroke Team had been successful plus pressure on beds and a desire to enable older people to return home and reduce the need for long term residential care.
Specialist nurse	LEAD CLINICIAN	Occupational Therapist
At home. ERP patients cared for in local community hospital until equipment installed at home	LOCATION	In patient's homes or in residential homes
9.00 - 17.00, Monday to Friday	AVAILABILITY OF SERVICE	9.00 - 17.00 (with District Nursing Evening Service covering out of hours). 7 days a week (skeleton service at weekends for essential work and emergencies.)
Open referral system	ACCESS TO THE SERVICE	Referral via letter, phone or fax by primary health care team, social services, hospital or self-referral (if patient already known to service).
Initial assessment by specialist nurse. Advice & information about stroke. Detailed assessments by relevant therapists. Multi-disciplinary goal setting and recording level of disability using FIM. Regular therapy aimed at clients goals within their home	CARE OFFERED	Physical rehabilitation and nursing needs.
Different packages of care provided - not time limited	TIME LIMITATION	6 weeks
Team decision in partnership with clients and carers	RESPONSIBILITY FOR DISCHARGE	Key clinician for that patient
55	NO. USING SERVICE	Up to 90
60 patients treated. 30 referrals, new assessments	NO. OVER PREVIOUS MONTH	112 new referrals
Above 17 years	AGE RANGE	65+
1.5 x Physio (1 x Superintendent: 0.5 x Senior I), 1.5 x OT Sen I, 0.5 x SaLT, 1.0 x Therapy Assistant, 1.0 x Specialist Neurology Nurse grade G, 1.0 x Secretary grade 4.	TEAM MEMBERS	Occupational Therapists Head III x1, Senior I x1, Senior II x 1; Physiotherapists Senior I x1.42, Senior II x 0.75; Nurses E x2, B x4
Evaluation at end of 3 year project - service became 'core' funded. Achieved National Award from the National Stroke Association, 1997. Team part of 3 year evaluation of community stroke services at Leeds University	MEASURED BY/EVALUATION	Peer audit – professionals (eg OTs)are sent out together to watch each other in their work. Observations are then discussed at one of the regular team meetings. Trust audit – paperwork/process audit.
Surveys show significant effect for clients & families/ carers. Outcome measures used ie. FIM, Barthel, Rivermead Mobility Index, Canadian Occ. Perf. Measure, Pam Enderby Scale, COOP, show positive outcome	IMPACT/OUTCOMES	Barthel audit tool is used both at the beginning and end of treatment by the team to assess improvement in activities of daily living.
Team too small to cope with the no. of referrals, espec. physio. Expansion to comm. rehab facility planned	LESSONS LEARNT/PLANS	Need good lines of communication with other services at planning stage.
Referral protocol, service leaflets. Evaluation reports	DOCUMENTATION AVAILABLE	Procedure documentation. Care pathways.
Miss Ruth Empson, Specialist Nurse, Community Stroke Team, Carshalton War Memorial Hospital, The Park, Carshalton, Surrey SM5 3DB Tel: 0181-669 7221	CONTACT	Jill Jackson, Clinical Support Manager, IC Services, Disability Resource Centre, Poynters Road, Dunstable LU5 4TP Tel: 01582 709021 Fax: 01582 709057

Community rehabilitation - home based

THANET HEALTH CARE TRUST (NHS 3RD WAVE TRUST)	*NAME OF NHS TRUST*
Elderly Rehabilitation Support Service	*NAME OF PROJECT/SCHEME*
Facilitate early discharge and improve rehab services	*PURPOSE OF SCHEME*
Links direct with Social Services	*MULTI-AGENCY INVOLVEMENT*
February 1998	*START DATE*
£158,000	*FUNDING*
To improve rehab services. To reduce bed days where appropriate	*REASON FOR INTRODUCTION*
At home	*LOCATION*
7.5 hours a day, 5 days a week	*AVAILABILITY OF SERVICE*
Referral through Trust	*ACCESS TO THE SERVICE*
Up to three visits per day depending on need. This may be additionally supported by Social Services involvement	*CARE OFFERED*
6 weeks	*TIME LIMITATION*
G grade nurse in conjunction with team	*RESPONSIBILITY FOR DISCHARGE*
Up to 35	*NO. USING SERVICE*
28	*NO. OVER PREVIOUS MONTH*
60-92	*AGE RANGE*
G grade nurse x 1, F x 1; Physio Snr I x 1; OT Snr I x 0.75, Dietician x 0.5; Rehab Support Workers x 3.85	*TEAM MEMBERS*
Currently Barthel, length of stay, bed days saved. Looking at alternatives to Barthel Score	*MEASURED BY/EVALUATION*
Difficult to measure. All patients have been treated successfully. Wards feel an impact re turnover – with relatively small numbers this does not show on any figures yet. However, patients treated are very positive about service.	*IMPACT/OUTCOMES*
Takes at least a year to see results. Support of higher management essential. More promotion would have been beneficial. Seeking funding to support cover for 5-10pm and at weekends.	*LESSONS LEARNT/PLANS*
Patient information leaflet	*DOCUMENTATION AVAILABLE*
Mark Clark, Co-ordinator Elderly Rehab, Devon House, St Peters Road, Margate, Kent CT9 4AN Tel: 01843 298533 (ansaphone) or 01843 225544 (switchboard). Available on pager.	*CONTACT*

Community rehabilitation - residential/day care

GREENWICH HEALTHCARE TRUST (IN ASSOCIATION WITH BUPA NURSING HOMES)	NAME OF NHS TRUST	COMMUNITY HEALTH SOUTH LONDON NHS TRUST
Intermediate Care Beds Scheme (The Bevan Unit)	NAME OF PROJECT/SCHEME	Lambeth Community Care Centre
To provide intensive nursing care & rehab for adults for a time limited period to optimise independence and enable patients to return home wherever possible. Targets people in the community & hosp. patients requiring rehab	PURPOSE OF SCHEME	To prevent institutionalisation and disability, facilitate early discharge and improve function.
The Management Board of unit includes reps from medicine (2x GP), SS, Trust, patients, HA, unit manager	MULTI-AGENCY INVOLVEMENT	Links with primary care, Social Services, and voluntary sector.
August 1997	START DATE	1985
Tomlinson funds to 31.3.99; Greenwich Healthcare Trust budget from 1.4.99	FUNDING	Health Authority
Difficult/distant access to local hospitals. Concern that many patients could avoid hospital admission if a local 'high care, low tech' facility was available. Opportunity for GPs to extend their role and offer a wider range of treatments in conjunction with nursing and therapy staff.	REASON FOR INTRODUCTION	Closure of 'local' district hospital. GP, CHC and Community initiative.
Two local GPs. Patients remain under the care of their GP. Consultant input when necessary.	LEAD CLINICIAN	Lead clinician in nursing, physio, OT, SaLT
Beds are leased from a BUPA nursing home	LOCATION	At community care centre where inpatient, day care and outpatient facilities are available
24 hours, 7 days a week	AVAILABILITY OF SERVICE	Varies for ward and day care
Only by referral from the patient's GP (even if in hospital). Referrals assessed by nurse manager to ensure that proper care and treatment can be provided.	ACCESS TO THE SERVICE	Majority by GP referral or through referral by SaLT/ chiropody/ dentist. Other services are all GP contracted. Any GP with practice wihin 5 miles can refer patients.
24 hour nursing care is available. General post-op rehab, wound management and assessment for social services.	CARE OFFERED	Nurse led ward – 20 beds, Day care, out-patients – OT, SaLT, physio, dentist, chiropody. Age 16+ rehab respite, palliative acute, assessment treatment.
Max 28 days (average LoS approx. 18 days)	TIME LIMITATION	Max expected LoS to ward = 28 days, otherwise none
The patient's GP, in consultation with the nurse manager	RESPONSIBILITY FOR DISCHARGE	Nursing staff
25 beds (current occupancy levels approx 95%) Approx. 40-45 admissions per month	NO. USING SERVICE NO. OVER PREVIOUS MONTH	Day:15 per day. OP: varies. In-patients: 20 Physio 200 new referrals. OT 25 new referrals. SALT 10 new referrals. Ward: 33 FCE, Day care, 7 new referrals
1.00 grade H nurse (nursing director); 3.00 grade F nurse; 4.0 grade E nurse; 2.0 grade B nurse (HCA), 6.00 grade A nurse (HCA), 2.0 nurse bank grade A; 1.0 physiotherapist (Senior II); 1.0 occupational therapist (Senior II); 0.2 dietician (Senior II); 0.2 speech and lang; 1.0 secretary, 0.8 screener assessor (social services)	TEAM MEMBERS	OT: 3; Sen I; Basic grade, assistant (A/CB). SALT: 2 33-35 x1, 24-28 x1. Ward nursing: Hx1, Fx2, Ex5, Dx3, Ax7. Day care: Ex1, A/C 4x1, Activities Co-ordinator. Dentist: x1, Dental Nurse x1. Physio: Super III 1.0, Sen I 1.0, Sen II 0.7, Assistant 0.5 (A/C 3), Basic grade 1.0. Chir 0.15
An external evaluation was undertaken by Greenwich University in 1998	MEASURED BY/EVALUATION	Outcome measures, Quality monitoring, FCE/occupancy. In-patient respite evaluation 1998 and 1999. Audits. Performance indicators. Satis. surveys.
Unit has been a success. High patient satisfaction; reduced hosp admissions, discharges accelerated. Occupancy rates near 95-100% (approx 40% cheaper than hospital bed)	IMPACT/OUTCOMES	Reduction in institutionalisation of elderly. Reduction in waiting list time for OPD's. Increased GP client /carer satisfaction.Reduction in DNA rate to OPD's. Prevents admission to acute hospital. Comm involvement and support. Highly valued. New Unit being built: April 2000.
Final Report Evaluating the Bevan IC Bed Unit (Sept 1998), Bamber Postance et al, Greenwich University	DOCUMENTATION AVAILABLE	Operational Policy. Currently updating centre leaflet. Staffing costs are available.
Ms Miriam Liew (Nurse Manager), The Bevan IC Beds Unit, Gallians View Nursing Home, 20 Pier Way, Thamesmead, London SE28 0EU Tel: 0181-854 2569 Fax: 0181-854 2544	CONTACT	Cathy Ingram, Service Manager, Lambeth Community Care Centre, Monkton Street, Kennington, London SE11 4TX Tel: 0171-582 5513 x217 Fax: 0171-735 0073

Community rehabilitation - residential/day care

SOUTHMEAD HEALTH TRUST, BRISTOL SOCIAL SERVICES DEPARTMENT, AVON HEALTH	NAME OF NHS TRUST	COMMUNITY HEALTH SHEFFIELD (CHS)
North Bristol Rehabilitation Centre	NAME OF PROJECT/SCHEME	Community Rehabilitation Unit (CRU)
To provide social rehabilitation for older people, to facilitate their return home.	PURPOSE OF SCHEME	The CRU provides a 'halfway house' between hospital and home environment. Each patient receives planned programme of rehab therapy aimed at achieving maximum function and independence
Social Services/Health	MULTI-AGENCY INVOLVEMENT	Partnership between CHS and private sector. Kersal Mount Nursing Home & Central Sheffield Univ Hospital
October 1998 – 7 beds April 1999 – Increase to 12 beds April 2000 – Increase to 20 beds	START DATE	November 1997
Joint funded with Avon Health for 3 years	FUNDING	Sheffield Health Authority.
To provide a wider range of options for older people to enable them to remain at home and prevent unnecessary admissions to residential/nursing care	REASON FOR INTRODUCTION	Reconfiguration of services previously based at Nether Edge Hospital.
Social services manager with OT/Physiotherapist support	LEAD CLINICIAN	Not known
Rehabilitation Centre	LOCATION	Community Rehabilitation Unit
24 hours, 7 days a week	AVAILABILITY OF SERVICE	24 hours, 7 days a week
Referrals can be made by post/fax to the Centre from health professionals (GPs, nurses, therapists) and social services	ACCESS TO THE SERVICE	Via 2 consultants based at Central Sheffield University Hospitals (Dr Anderson and Dr Hendra).
OT and Physio draw up individual rehabilitation programmes. Care Officers work with service users and provide hands-on care as necessary. Medical input provided by GPs and District Nurses.	CARE OFFERED	Multi-disciplinary rehabilitation to elderly patients residing in the south of the city.
Usually 6 week programme – can be less	TIME LIMITATION	22 weeks
Centre Manager	RESPONSIBILITY FOR DISCHARGE	Consultants
12 as of April 1999	NO. USING SERVICE	20
7 in March 1999	NO. OVER PREVIOUS MONTH	20
65-95	AGE RANGE	65+, average 85
1 Centre Manager, 2 Assistant Centre Managers, 5.3 Care Officers, 2 Night Care Assistants, 0.5 Admin Assistant, 2.7 Domestics, 1 Cook. 1 OT and 1 Physio – Health Service employees.	TEAM MEMBERS	Nursing staff provided by nursing home ratio 1:4, 2 x physios II, 1.6 x OT II, 4 x therapy assistants, 1 x nursing rehab co-ordinator, 0.5 x SW, 1 x admin and clerical grade II, sessional member speech and language therapy, dietetics, psychology, podiatry, GP clinical assistants.
4 week review. Follow up at 3, 6 and 9 months. Full evaluation of 1st year in October 1999 when significant number of service users have been discharged. Also measuring services needed after discharge in comparison with those needed pre-admission.	MEASURED BY/EVALUATION	Barthel index. Elderly mobility scale. Clinical Audit. Research and Evaluation.
Referrals steadily increasing as professionals become aware of services. Need to be operating for one year to be able to evaluate the outcome for a significant number of people.	IMPACT/OUTCOMES	Contributes to wider strategy for rehabilitation within Sheffield an standardisation of Therapy Outcome measures across Sheffield. Actively encourages a multidisciplinary model of rehab and clinical intervention.
Issues paper for future due in May 1999	DOCUMENTATION AVAILABLE	Annual Report 1997
Nikki Cole, Team Manager, Welsman, Bishop Street, St Pauls, Bristol, BS2 9JA Tel: 0117-9036734 Fax: 0117 9036739; Diane Jepson, Centre Manager, NBRC, c/o Hazelbrook, 20 Ellesworth Road, Henbury, Bristol, BS10 7EH Tel: 0117-959 0752	CONTACT	Pauline Bramley, Therapy Manager, CHS, Fulwood House, Fulwood Road, Sheffield

Community rehabilitation - residential/day care

COMMUNITY HEALTH SHEFFIELD	NAME OF NHS TRUST	LIVERPOOL HEALTH AUTHORITY
Assessment and Rehabilitation Centre (ARC)	NAME OF PROJECT/SCHEME	Joint Rehabilitation Scheme
Rehabilitation and assessment unit for older people, with 40 places available each day. Aims to maintain people in the community and so prevent admission. To continue care after discharge from hospital or Community Rehab Team. To offer rehabilitation to patients following deterioration in physical and functional ability.	PURPOSE OF SCHEME	To provide rehabilitation. To increase number of patients able to return home and reduce number of nursing home placements.
Nurses. Physio. OT. Psychology. Dietitian. Dental. Chiropody. Medical	MULTI-AGENCY INVOLVEMENT	Acute Trust. Community Trust. Social Services. GPs.
1974. Service reviewed 1995	START DATE	May 1998
CHS Trust, through Sheffield Health Authority	FUNDING	Joint finance.
Long established, but service provision renewed as the focus of care moved into the community.	REASON FOR INTRODUCTION	Response to winter pressures and high number of nursing home placements in city.
Centre within a former hospital	LOCATION	Rehab unit within social services residential care home. Follow up care for 4-6 weeks within patients' homes.
8.00 to 17.30, Monday to Friday	AVAILABILITY OF SERVICE	24 hours, 7 days a week
Through referral from any health or social care worker	ACCESS TO THE SERVICE	Referral from wards via social worker
Multidisciplinary assessment and programme of rehabilitation	CARE OFFERED	Short term rehab in residential care setting based on social model
No	TIME LIMITATION	4-6 weeks
Team decision	RESPONSIBILITY FOR DISCHARGE	Co-ordinator following MDT decision
40 places a day	NO. USING SERVICE	5
Total number of attendances = 632	NO. OVER PREVIOUS MONTH	8
Approx 15% under 65 years, 85% over 65 years	AGE RANGE	65+
Nursing: 1.0 G grade, 1.0 F grade, 1.7 E grade, 4.57 D grade, 4.24 A grade. Housekeeper 1.86 scale B. PT: 1.0 Sen I, 2.2 Sen II, 1.0 Asst. OT: 1.0 Sen I, 1.0 Sen II, 1.0 basic grade, 1.0 Ass. Dr: 0.45. Psychology: 0.3 Consultant Clinical. Consultant: 0.2. Speech & language therapists: 0.4 specialist, 0.6 basic grade	TEAM MEMBERS	Full time Co-ordinator, 6.5 WTE Carers, Physiotherapy 0.3, Occupational Therapy 0.3.
Post course evaluations and 6 month reviews. Reflective practice – critical incidents. Evaluations following development days (yearly). Patient Satisfaction Questionnaires	MEASURED BY/EVALUATION	Full evaluation being developed
ARC strategy for the next year developed at Unit Development Day	IMPACT/OUTCOMES	Occupancy 89% 6 months Sept-March. 80% patients returned home. 20% patients to nursing/res care. Average LoS 33 days.
As client needs change, the service provision has to be reviewed regularly	LESSONS LEARNT/PLANS	Need to build firm networks and engage front line staff early on. Expansion of scheme.
Service provision. Development Day Report. Patient information leaflet.	DOCUMENTATION AVAILABLE	
Sister Maggie Howsley, Manager, Assessment and Rehabilitation Centre, Michael Carlisle Centre, Nether Edge Hospital, Osborne Road, Sheffield S11 9BL Tel: 0114-271 6571 Fax: 0114-271 6574	CONTACT	John Davies, The Rehabilitation Unit, Leighton Dene, Long Lane, Liverpool, L9 9DW

Community rehabilitation - residential/day care

NORTHERN BIRMINGHAM COMMUNITY NHS TRUST	*NAME OF NHS TRUST*
Richard Lawn Rehabilitation Service	*NAME OF PROJECT/SCHEME*
To facilitate early discharge from hospital. To prevent inappropriate permanent admission to residential care. To provide a rehabilitation programme. To enable older people to remain as independent as possible living in their own homes.	*PURPOSE OF SCHEME*
Multi-agency team. Nurses, physiotherapist, occupational therapist, speech and language therapists, GPs, geriatricians, podiatrists, dietitians, care assistants, other multi agency team members. Social workers	*MULTI-AGENCY INVOLVEMENT*
September 1998	*START DATE*
Joint Health and Social Services funding	*FUNDING*
Identified need for rehabilitation programme for older people in the inner city area of Ladywood Birmingham, for strokes, falls, fractures or orthopaedic intervention.	*REASON FOR INTRODUCTION*
Clinical nurse specialist	*LEAD CLINICIAN*
Care for people in a community setting (residentiual home) with follow up care provided in people's homes	*LOCATION*
24 hours, 7 days a week	*AVAILABILITY OF SERVICE*
Discharge from hospital wards City Hospital Birmingham. Discharge from A&E Dept. Access via community referrals from GPs, DNs, social workers. Referrals will be accepted from any sources	*ACCESS TO THE SERVICE*
Health and social care – rehab in all areas of physical, psychological/emotional, social care to enable people to return to their own homes as independent as possible	*CARE OFFERED*
Residential short term stay for up to 8 weeks. Outreach units for up to 8 months	*TIME LIMITATION*
The rehabilitation team in collaboration with the clients and carers	*RESPONSIBILITY FOR DISCHARGE*
10 bedded unit	*NO. USING SERVICE*
8 (capacity for 10)	*NO. OVER PREVIOUS MONTH*
68-89 years	*AGE RANGE*
RGN xH grade x 1; RGN xG grade x 1; RGN E grade x 5; physiotherapist x 0.7; OT x 0.3; speech and language therapist x 0.3; social worker x 0.5; care assistants x 9; GP cover 24 hours a day; dietitian sessional basis, podiatrist sessional basis	*TEAM MEMBERS*
Evaluation of service being undertaken by team at Keele University	*MEASURED BY/EVALUATION*
Good impact and outcome measures are being obtained from the rehabilitation intervention and evaluation programme	*IMPACT/OUTCOMES*
Positive lessons learnt from inter-agency working. Importance of team working and development	*LESSONS LEARNT/PLANS*
Inter-agency/interdisc. documentation being developed	*DOCUMENTATION AVAILABLE*
Annette Hanny, Rehabilitation Manager and Sylvia Harvey, Clinical Nurse Specialist, Richard Lawn Rehabilitation Service, Ladywood, Birmingham B16 8EB Tel: 0121-236 8365 Fax: 0121-236 2364	*CONTACT*

Hospital at Home

COMMUNITY HEALTH SHEFFIELD (CHS)	*NAME OF NHS TRUST*	**COMMUNITY HEALTH SHEFFIELD (CHS)**
Intensive Home Nursing Service for terminally ill adults and the elderly	*NAME OF PROJECT/SCHEME*	Intensive Home Nursing Service – Hospital at Home with Therapy Services for the over 65s
To care for terminally patients at home, allowing them to die at home.	*PURPOSE OF SCHEME*	To prevent hospital admission by offering a home based package of care for a maximum of 7 days
Complements District Nursing Service and Macmillan Support Team.	*MULTI-AGENCY INVOLVEMENT*	Nursing. Occupational therapy. Physiotherapy. Pharmacy services.
1994	*START DATE*	Piloted 1993. Commenced 1994. City wide 1996.
Sheffield Health Authority.	*FUNDING*	Sheffield Health Authority. Approximately £900,00 per annum.
To offer dying patients a choice of where to die and offer support to carers	*REASON FOR INTRODUCTION*	
	LEAD CLINICIAN	The GP retains medical responsibility and manages medical care
Home based	*LOCATION*	In people's homes
24 hours, 7 days a week.	*AVAILABILITY OF SERVICE*	24 hours, 7 days a week
Via the Co-ordinator on duty 9.00 to 22.00 or ringing the office between 8.00 and 18.00 Mon-Fri or 8.00 to 12.00 Sat, Sun and Bank Holidays.	*ACCESS TO THE SERVICE*	Via a Co-ordinator (a registered nurse) on duty or ringing the office between 8.00 and 18.00 Mon-Fri; 8.00 to 12.00 Sat, Sun and Bank Holidays. No self referrals.
Up to 24 hour nursing care at home during the last week of life. For the last month of life may have a night auxiliary every night to give care and support the family/ carers.	*CARE OFFERED*	Up to 24 hour nursing care at home with physiotherapy and occupational therapy services if required.
Approximately last week of life for 24 hour care	*TIME LIMITATION*	Maximum 7 days
Co-ordinators	*RESPONSIBILITY FOR DISCHARGE*	Co-ordinator
N/A	*NO. USING SERVICE*	10
N/A	*NO. OVER PREVIOUS MONTH*	
N/A	*AGE RANGE*	65 years and over
1.92 x G grade co-ordinator; 2 x F grade co-ordinators; 45.09 x B grade auxiliaries; 1.07 x clerical support	*TEAM MEMBERS*	1.92 x G grade co-ordinators; 2 x F grade co-ordinators; 45.09 x B grade auxiliaries; 1.07 x clerical support.
Evaluated by ScHARR, Sheffield University	*MEASURED BY/EVALUATION*	Evaluated by ScHARR, Sheffield University
Allowing patient a choice – providing a seamless service for dying patients.	*IMPACT/OUTCOMES*	Preventing hospital admissions. Allowing patients to remain at home in familiar surroundings and alleviating the distress and confusion caused by hospital admission.
Angela Barrowclough & Helen Clark, Co-ordinators, Intensive Home Nursing Services, Woodhouse Clinic, 3 Skelton Lane, Sheffield, S13 7LY Tel: 0114 254 8760 Fax: 0114 269 1916	*CONTACT*	Angela Barrowclough, Co-ordinator Intensive Home Nusrsing Service, Woodhouse Clinic, 3 Skelton Lane, Sheffield S13 7LY Tel: 0114-254 8760 Fax: 0114-269 1916

Hospital at Home

MERTON AND SUTTON COMMUNITY NHS TRUST	NAME OF NHS TRUST	LEEDS COMMUNITY AND MENTAL HEALTH TRUST
Community Hospital at Home	NAME OF PROJECT/SCHEME	Hospital at Home
To prevent inappropriate acute hospital admission. To facilitate early/timely discharge.	PURPOSE OF SCHEME	To facilitate early discharge. To prevent hospital admission.
Liaise closely with GP, district nurses, social service and voluntary services as appropriate.	MULTI-AGENCY INVOLVEMENT	Close liaison with local social services.
September 1993	START DATE	Scheme has been running for several years. Hospital at Home team started November 1994.
£418,000 pa and Challenge Fund monies recurring. Health Authority (approx. £235,000). Local TPP contract (£183,000).	FUNDING	Leeds Community and Mental Health Trust (£134,125). Care of elderly department at Leeds General Infirmary (£160,000). Total has been boosted in recent years with winter pressures monies.
Local and national emphasis on care in the community. Pressure on community services and acute services.	REASON FOR INTRODUCTION	To offer rehabilitation to over 65s at home and to prevent an unnecessary hospital admission. Closure of local elderly care beds has led to more services being provided in community settings.
Nurse led service.	LEAD CLINICIAN	Overall management of the team from clinical leader.
At home	LOCATION	At home.
24 hours, 7 days a week	AVAILABILITY OF SERVICE	8.30 - 22.00, 7 days a week,.
Either by telephone during office hours or on call bleep. Will take referrals from other health professionals and social sercices. Occasionally patients self-refer.	ACCESS TO THE SERVICE	Open referral system, via DN, GP, Social Services, carers and liaison sister based in the hospital.
Complete packages of nursing and social care with therapy as required. Emphasis is usually on rehabilitation	CARE OFFERED	Personal care. Rehabilitation – physio (mobility), OT. Nursing care eg. medication, wound care etc.
Aim is for 2 weeks on the scheme, but longer episodes of care are available.	TIME LIMITATION	4-6 weeks
Named nurse/team leader in collaboration with others involved in care	RESPONSIBILITY FOR DISCHARGE	Physiotherapists, occupational therapists or nurses.
12-24 depending on dependency	NO. USING SERVICE	25 or 35 when winter pressures money available.
56	NO. OVER PREVIOUS MONTH	60
16-97	AGE RANGE	65+, most patients are in the 70s, 80s.
H grade 1.0, G grade 1.6, F grade 1.0, E grade 3.27, D grade 4.7, B grade 7.2, Physiotherapist Sen I 1.74, OT 0,5 (vacant), A&C 1.2.	TEAM MEMBERS	1x H nurse, 1x G nurse, 0.25 x G nurse, 1x E nurse, 1x OT, 1.5x Senior I Physio, 5x 1 HSW, 9x 0.53 HSW, 2x Admin staff (1.13).
Barthel index. Patient satisfaction. Readmission rates. Clinical review group with TPP patients. Evaluation exercise planned for later this year.	MEASURED BY/EVALUATION	Quarterly Patient Charter monitoring. User/carer satis.surveys.Data on patients referred, discharged, length of time in scheme, total patients accepted on scheme collected monthly for Leeds General Infirmary.
Generally closer working and integration between services. Reduction in some emergency admissions.	IMPACT/OUTCOMES	
Extend use of service by other GPs/PCGs. Development of care pathways. Close integration with other services.	LESSONS LEARNT/PLANS	Leeds is in the process of being reconfigured regarding all elderly care services. Hospital beds are being closed so that care can be given in the community by Hospital at Home, intensive home treatment, or spot purchasing of nursing home bed where appropriate. Future services now community based, but acute beds available if required.
Descriptive information about scheme eg. patient leaflets.	DOCUMENTATION AVAILABLE	Information leaflets about the scheme.
Eileen Clark, Co-ordinator, Community Hospital at Home, Carshalton War Memorial Hospital, The Park, Carshalton, Surrey SM5 3DB Tel: 0181-773 1030 Fax: 0181-669 3390	CONTACT	Pamela Young, Clinical Leader, Hospital at Home, Kirkstall Health Centre, Morris Lane, Leeds LS5 3DB Tel: 0113-295 1524 Fax: 0113-295 1161

Hospital at Home

LEICESTERSHIRE AND RUTLAND HEALTHCARE NHS TRUST (FORMERLY FOSSE HEALTH TRUST – COMMUNITY)	*NAME OF NHS TRUST*	FRENCHAY NHS TRUST – COMBINED ACUTE & COMMUNITY
Hospital at Home	*NAME OF PROJECT/SCHEME*	Hospital at Home
To prevent hospital admission	*PURPOSE OF SCHEME*	Facilitate early discharge. Prevention of admission.
Joint working with social services during the winter period	*MULTI-AGENCY INVOLVEMENT*	Plans to develop social rehabilitation within the team in conjunction with social services.
January 1994	*START DATE*	April 1994
Initially City Challenge money and then Leicestershire Health Authority.	*FUNDING*	Recurring funding which has been temporarily increased from winter pressures monies.
To reduce the number of patients being admitted to hospital to die and ease pressure on acute hospitals. No GP beds available in City of Leicester.	*REASON FOR INTRODUCTION*	Belief that more could be done in the community. Extra funding gave opportunity to try.
GPs maintain medical responsibility for patients	*LEAD CLINICIAN*	Team is led by a district nurse.
In people's homes	*LOCATION*	At home.
24 hours, 7 days a week.	*AVAILABILITY OF SERVICE*	8.30 to 22.00; 7 days a week (open 8.30-17.00 for referrals).
By referral from GP to a central Bed Bureau and then an assessment by Hospital at Home within two hours.	*ACCESS TO THE SERVICE*	Early discharge: referral from member of multidisciplinary team at the hospital. Patient assessed while still on ward. Prevention of admission: referral from GP, A&E staff member of PHCT with GP consent. Team has widely publicised telephone number.
Up to 24 hours care a day. Multidisciplinary care. Nurses, physiotherapists, occupational therapists – supported by generic health care assistants.	*CARE OFFERED*	Multi/inter-disciplinary rehabilitation.
Maximum 14 days	*TIME LIMITATION*	Maximum 28 days.
The named nurse, after consulting with the multidisciplinary team and the GP.	*RESPONSIBILITY FOR DISCHARGE*	Key professional responsible for care following discussion with team.
Fluctuates between 5 and 14 (average 8)	*NO. USING SERVICE*	30
December 98 = 49, January 99 = 34	*NO. OVER PREVIOUS MONTH*	78 new referrals in Jan. 1999.
Hospital at Home accepts patients from 16 years of age – but average age is 85 years.	*AGE RANGE*	18+
Project Manager H grade 0.8; G grade sister x 1.00; B grade generic H.C.W x 11.00; Sen I occupational therapist x 1.00; secretary/administrator x 1.00; E grade named nurses x 9.00; Sen I physiotherapist x 1.00	*TEAM MEMBERS*	G grade district nurse x 1; F grade nurse x 1; E grade nurse x 1.75; B grade nurse x 2.31, Senior I physiotherapist x 0.83; Senior I occupational therapist x 0.69. (More therapy hours as required from WP monies).
Randomised Controlled Trial (RCT) undertaken by Dept of General Practice, Leicester University(Dr Andrew Wilson, Hilda Parker, Alison Wynn).To be published in BMJ	*MEASURED BY/EVALUATION*	RCT by Department Social Medicine, Bristol University. Refs: 'Effectiveness and acceptability of early discharge at home schemes', BMJ, 13 June 1998, Vol. 316, pp 1796-1801; and 'Cost minimisation analysis', BMJ, 13 June 1998, Vol. 316, pp 1802-1806.
For patients referred to HAH during the trial period: HAH appears to provide safe alternative to hosp admis. LoS significantly shorter in HAH compared to hospital. HAH does not confer a greater risk of re-admission or increased use of community services. Patients in HAH were more satisfied with care. HAH episode costs were cheaper than hospital.	*IMPACT/OUTCOMES*	Developing system with in-house computer department to measure number of bed days saved. Headlines from RCT – HAH appears to be cost-effective, outcome neutral and more popular with patients, though some difficulties in comparing scheme costs with hospital costs.
Leaflets in English, Gugarati & Punjabi. In press BMJ article	*DOCUMENTATION AVAILABLE*	
Mrs J Bergstrom, Acting Manager, Hospital at Home, New Parks Health Centre, St Oswald Road, Leicester LE3 6RJ Tel: 0116 2871291 Fax: 0116 287 5312	*CONTACT*	Mary-Anne Darlow, Hospital at Home Co-ordinator, Downend Clinic, Buckingham Gardens, BS16 5TW Tel: 0117 9566025 Fax: 0117 9561907

Hospital at Home

BEDFORDSHIRE AND LUTON COMMUNITY NHS TRUST	*NAME OF NHS TRUST*
Hospital at Home	*NAME OF PROJECT/SCHEME*
To enable patients to be discharged home early after surgery	*PURPOSE OF SCHEME*
Luton and Dunstable Hospital	*MULTI-AGENCY INVOLVEMENT*
1995	*START DATE*
Bedfordshire Health Authority, Winter Pressures Monies, Challenge Fund. Total: £142,950	*FUNDING*
To reduce pressure on acute beds at the hospital	*REASON FOR INTRODUCTION*
A nurse	*LEAD CLINICIAN*
In patient's own home	*LOCATION*
24 hours, 7 days a week	*AVAILABILITY OF SERVICE*
By referral to Hospital at Home team from Consultant by phone/fax. Good liaison with hospital staff.	*ACCESS TO THE SERVICE*
Post-operative care. Physiotherapy	*CARE OFFERED*
No time limit. However, typically care is provided for the following number of post-operative days: gynaecological surgery 5 days; orthopaedic surgery 10-14 days; breast surgery 10 days	*TIME LIMITATION*
The last professional to see the patient	*RESPONSIBILITY FOR DISCHARGE*
Between 10-15	*NO. USING SERVICE*
40	*NO. OVER PREVIOUS MONTH*
16-80	*AGE RANGE*
Nurses 1.7 + Bank; physiotherapist 0.5; Team Assistant 0.5	*TEAM MEMBERS*
Peer Audit	*MEASURED BY/EVALUATION*
Pathways of care are constantly reviewed with the hospital staff and the consultant so as to ensure that they remain up to date with the latest treatments.	*IMPACT/OUTCOMES*
To extend the Hospital at Home service to other suitable conditions	*LESSONS LEARNT/PLANS*
Integrated Care Pathway and management reports	*DOCUMENTATION AVAILABLE*
Jill Jackson, Clinical Support Manager, Intermediate Care Services, Disability Resource Centre, Poynters Road, Dunstable LU5 4TP Tel: 01582 709 021 Fax: 01582 709057	*CONTACT*

Children's services

NAME OF NHS TRUST	HOMERTON HOSPITAL NHS TRUST	MANCUNIAN COMMUNITY HEALTH NHS TRUST
NAME OF PROJECT/SCHEME	Geffrye Children's Unit (Paediatric Ambulatory Care Centre)	Community Paediatric Nurse in an A&E setting.
PURPOSE OF SCHEME	To minimise hospital admissions for children and to reduce lengths of stay. To bridge the gap between primary and secondary children's services.	To prevent inappropriate admission to hospital. To increase care in the community. To facilitate early discharge.
MULTI AGENCY INVOLVEMENT	Close links with Community Trust, GP's, Social Services.	Manchester Children's Hospital NHS Trust, Mancunian Community Health NHS Trust.
START DATE	Interim Unit – 24 September 1998. New unit due to open – June/July 1999.	November 1998
FUNDING	£2.3 million in capital funding to develop ambulatory paediatrics at the Homerton, following the closure of Queen Elizabeth Hospital for Children.	3 year transitional funding from Health Authority.
REASON FOR INTRODUCTION	Review of children's services across East London. Opportunity to change pattern of paediatric services. Evidence that children could be managed at home and did not like being in hospital	To enable more children to be cared for in their own environment. To develop the community service in preparation for the reconfiguration of children's services in Manchester.
LEAD CLINICIAN	2 lead clinicians - 1 nurse, 1 paediatric consultant	G grade nurse.
LOCATION	Care can be provided for up to 24 hours in hospital and up to 2 weeks at home with hospital overnight stay.	In patient's home.
AVAILABILITY OF SERVICE	24 hours, 7 days a week	12.00 - 20.00 in A&E. Comm. 8.30- 22.00 daily.
ACCESS TO THE SERVICE	Via Paediatric A&E Department. Via GP Rapid Referral Clinic (held daily). Self-referral via telephone. Transfer from other hospital.	Anyone can refer (GPs, A & E Dept. etc) by letter or phone. In A&E setting, the child has joint assessment for care in community. If applicable, referred to Children's Community Nursing Service for continuing care.
CARE OFFERED	General paediatric care in a setting appropriate to the child's needs. This may be either: 24 hours short stay; Assessment Area; Out patients; Hospital-at-Home.	Advice to parents about medication, treatment and reassessment of conditions to ensure patient continues to be suitable for home based care.
TIME LIMITATION	Acute care only (ie. 24 hours hospital; 2 weeks home)	No time limits.
RESPONSIBILITY FOR DISCHARGE	Paediatric medical staff and paed. nurse practitioners	Each RGN paediatric nurse.
NO. USING SERVICE	1-20	Approximately 4 per day – fluctuates.
NO. OVER PREVIOUS MONTH		20 – fluctuates
AGE RANGE	0-16 years	0-16 years
TEAM MEMBERS	Large multi-disciplinary team including nurse practitioners, a nurse lecturer practitioner, consultant and middle grade doctors, social workers, dieticians and family workers (play specialists)	Children's Community Nursing Team – City Wide. G grade 2.8, E grade 5.8, B grade 1.5, 1.8 G grade rotate into A&E Booth Hall, 4.3 E rotate into A&E Booth Hall
MEASURED BY/EVALUATION	Care given via Multi-disciplinary Integrated Care Pathways (approx.100) - analysed weekly. Unit hopes to employ researcher/lecturer for evaluation	Consumer evaluation on discharge. Follow up questionnaire after 6 weeks. Professional views to be sought after 6 months via an audit process, comparison pre and post service.
IMPACT/OUTCOMES	Paediatric Clinical Governance Group meets every 6 weeks to analyse the impact. Expected health outcomes achieved and children/ families give positive feedback.	Better quality of care provided for children who previously received no service. Increased appreciation of roles though working together with common aim.
LESSONS LEARNT/PLANS	Due to almost double the service with move into new building in a few months. Plan to develop the role of the Paediatric Nurse Practitioner and Hospital-at-Home	Extending to other conditions, looking at seasonal variations and problems, and to other A&E departments.
DOCUMENTATION AVAILABLE	Integrated Care Pathways to be published later this year	Protocols. Information and advice sheets.
CONTACT	Louise Burke, Senior Nurse, Paediatrics & SCBU, Homerton Hospital NHS Trust, Homerton Row, London E9 6SR Tel: 0181-510 5555 Fax: 0181-510 7875	Mrs Peggy Keating, Children's CNT Manager, Brunswick Health Centre, Hartfield Close, Chorlton on Medlock, Manchester M13 9YA Tel: 0161 273 4901

Children's services

MANCUNIAN COMMUNITY HEALTH NHS TRUST	*NAME OF NHS TRUST*	MANCUNIAN COMMUNITY HEALTH NHS TRUST
Children's Community Nurses based at Children's A&E Department, Booth Hall Children's Hospital	*NAME OF PROJECT/SCHEME*	Children's Asthma Centre
To prevent unnecessary hospital admissions. To offer a better quality follow up service for children attending A&E. To have strategies in place for the major changes	*PURPOSE OF SCHEME*	To provide education, advice and support to children with asthma and their families. To promote self-management in asthma care.
	MULTI-AGENCY INVOLVEMENT	Acute Trust
	START DATE	Has been running since 1994
Manchester HA funded as part of transitional arrangements for reconfiguration of local paediatric services	*FUNDING*	
In the light of future changes to children's services in the Manchester hospitals, a new service was developed by the Children's Community Nursing Team (CCNT). Extra funding from HA enabled expansion of existing CCNT, with extended working day and an experienced CCN to be based in A&E department for up to 20.00 hours.	*REASON FOR INTRODUCTION*	To provide specialist centre.
Community paediatrician, joint appointment by acute and community Trusts	*LEAD CLINICIAN*	
A & E and then home	*LOCATION*	Nurses provide clinic (drop in) at Asthma Centre. Otherwise care is provided in patients' homes.
Flexible	*AVAILABILITY OF SERVICE*	Consultant physician monthly clinic (with 2 staff grade doctors). Specialist nurses provide weekly clinic on asthma management. Centre: 8.30 - 17.00, 5 days
Via A & E	*ACCESS TO THE SERVICE*	Open referral system.
Child and family assessed jointly by the Children's Community Nurse in A&Eand hospital medical and nursing staff, for suitability for home care. On discharge child and family referred to Community Nurses for follow up. Reassessment by the Community Nurse can take place at home within 2 hours of discharge from A&E and can be continued for as long as necessary. Most common conditions treated - bronchitis, asthma, sprains, falls, croup, pyrexia, UTI, febrile convulsions etc.	*CARE OFFERED*	A structured educational programme is adapted to suit each individual child and their family. Parents can contact the centre by telephone for continued advice and support Home visits, nurse-led drop-in clinics and doctor/nurse clinics are available. The centre acts as a resource for other health professionals particularly HVs and school nurses to gain information and advice. Training for health professionals and carers of children with asthma, eg. school staff, childminders.
	TIME LIMITATION	None.
Nurses	*RESPONSIBILITY FOR DISCHARGE*	
Typically patients are young babies or children up to 5 years. Asthmatics - up to 16 years	*PATIENT PROFILE*	
5 nominated members of the Children's Community Nursing Team work in the A&E department on a rotational basis. These are supported by the remainder of the Children's Community Nursing Team members.	*TEAM MEMBERS*	2 Asthma Nurse Specialists. 1 Consultant paediatrician. 1 Associate specialist in child health. 1 staff grade Community Paediatrician. 1 Secretary.
Has prevented hospital admissions	*OUTCOMES*	Research on drop-in clinic showed positive results for children and families. Centre has played a major role in joint initiative between the Mancunian Community Health NHS Trust and the Manchester Education Authority. Schools project aimed to improve the approach to asthma care in schools. Project audited over 1 year - results have shown an improvement in the management of asthma.
Planned write up of scheme	*DOCUMENTATION AVAILABLE*	
Mrs Val Smith, Nurse & Special Projects Co-ordinator, Children & Young People's Directorate, Mancunian Community Health NHS Trust, Mauldeth House, Mauldeth Road West, Chorlton, Manchester M21 7RL Tel: 0161-958 4124 Fax: 0161-958 4122	*CONTACT*	Mrs Val Smith, Nurse & Special Projects Co-ordinator, Children & Young People's Directorate, Mancunian Community Health NHS Trust, Mauldeth House, Mauldeth Road West, Chorlton, Manchester M21 7RL Tel: 0161-958 4124 Fax: 0161-958 4122

Nurse-led in-patient

NAME OF NHS TRUST	NORTH BRISTOL HEALTH SERVICE NHS TRUST	SOUTH TEES ACUTE HOSPITALS NHS TRUST
NAME OF PROJECT/SCHEME	Nurse-led intermediate care ward (Malvern Ward)	Interim Care Ward – nurse led
PURPOSE OF SCHEME	To relieve pressure on acute wards (mainly medicine). To allow more time for in-depth discharge planning	To take patients who are medically fit for discharge but whose discharge is delayed.
MULTI-AGENCY INVOLVEMENT	Nurse-led ward in general hospital. Hospital-based SW	A part-time social worker is attached to the ward.
START DATE	September 1997	December 1998
FUNDING	Southmead Health Services NHS Trust - 20 beds by Medical Directorate, 4 beds by Surgical Directorate.	No additional identified funding. Part of contract with Tees Health and Division of Medicine.
REASON FOR INTRODUCTION	Ongoing pressure on acute medical wards. Need to improve on discharge planning and outcomes for elderly patients, in particular.	Delayed discharges restricting the ability to admit medical emergencies. To further the role and the expertise for staff both qualified and unqualified in nurse-led care.
LEAD CLINICIAN	Ward manager/sister leads team of nurses and is responsible for overseeing patient care and co-ordination of discharge planning.	Nurses manage care. Patients remain under the care of the original consultant until discharge but will not usually see that consultant again during their stay in interim care.
LOCATION	Up-graded ward on main hospital site	Hospital ward.
AVAILABILITY OF SERVICE	24 hours, 7 days a week	24 hours, 7 days a week.
ACCESS TO THE SERVICE	From acute wards and via A&E. Patients assessed against agreed protocol criteria. Must be 'medically fit' for discharge.	Consultant referral to ward manager. It must be documented that patients are medically fit for discharge as medical cover for the ward is based on an as and when required rule.
CARE OFFERED	Nursing care. Limited rehabilitation from occupational therapist and Physio. (Difficult to transfer to rehab department for therapy due to location.)	Nursing care. Staff continue to promote independence and rehabilitation. Rehabilitation programmes should have been completed prior to admission to the ward as there are no attached therapy staff. Physiotherapy & OT can be assessed for individuals if required.
TIME LIMITATION	None, but expectation is that most patients will be discharged within a few weeks. Not a long-stay facility.	No
RESPONSIBILITY FOR DISCHARGE	Ward manager/sister, in consultation with social workers and Care Management Facilitator.	The ward manager who is lead sister.
NO. USING SERVICE	Maximum 24	20
NO. OVER PREVIOUS MONTH		42
AGE RANGE	Few under 65, most 75+ (significant number are 85+)	61 years +
TEAM MEMBERS	Health care assistants A 9.9 and B 3.06;staff nurse D 1.4; staff nurse E 6.46; staff nurse F 1.0; sister G 1.0; receptionist A&C grade 2 1.0.	1 x G grade sister; 7 x E grade staff nurses (3 of whom are part-time); 17 x 3A grade health care assistants (12 of whom are part-time).
MEASURED BY/EVALUATION	Analysis of monthly statistics	Report from experiences of ward supported the ethos of nurse-led care with benefits for patients and carers. Patient/Carer questionnaire has been developed.
IMPACT/OUTCOMES	Saving of acute bed days. Greater number of patients returning to own homes with community 'packages of care' than would otherwise have been the case. Potentially fewer residential/nursing home placements.	Releases much needed acute medical beds. More time and quieter atmosphere for patients promoting further recovery. Carers feel better supported in their decisions about future care. Opportunities for patients to visit residential/nursing homes prior to placement.
LESSONS LEARNT/PLANS	Patients tend to have very heavy nursing care needs. Need for a high level of continued social work input if patients are not to become 'stuck'. Need for community nursing and Care Management Facilitator input.	
DOCUMENTATION AVAILABLE	Monthly and annual statistics regarding prolonged patient stays. Bed usage. Destination on discharge.	Policy document.
CONTACT	Margaret Ruse, Specialist Nurse, Care Management, Nursing Directorate, Beaufort House, Southmead Hospital, Westbury-on-Trym, Bristol BS10 5NB Tel: 0117-950 5050 x3298 Fax: 0117-959 5589	Mrs Sue Dove, Discharge Co-ordinator, Division of Medicine, South Cleveland Hospital, Marton Road, Middlesbrough, Cleveland TS4 3BW Tel: 01642 850850 x3030 Fax: 01642 854748

Nurse-led in-patient

NAME OF NHS TRUST	DONCASTER HEALTHCARE NHS TRUST	GEORGE ELIOT HOSPITAL NHS TRUST (ACUTE TRUST)
NAME OF PROJECT/SCHEME	Recuperative Care Ward	Half Way Home
PURPOSE OF SCHEME	To provide recuperative care services whilst preparing and implementing packages of care for discharge for older highly dependent people	To facilitate timely, appropriate discharge for patients requiring community continuing care.
MULTI-AGENCY INVOLVEMENT	Acute and Community Trusts in Doncaster and Social Services Directorate	Nurses, doctors, social workers, occupational therapists, physiotherapists, psychologists.
START DATE	December 1997	July 1995
FUNDING	£240,000 from Doncaster Health Authority - originally funded through winter pressures monies	Joint HA and Social Service although HA is nominated purchaser.
REASON FOR INTRODUCTION	Initially to assist in winter emergency planning but recurrently funded due to success of scheme	To reduce bed blocking and to prevent readmission as a result of inappropriate discharge package.
LEAD CLINICIAN	Senior sister co-ordinates service, consultant physician in terms of discharge	Nurse/social worker.
LOCATION	Hospital ward	A refurbished 28 bedded ward.
AVAILABILITY OF SERVICE	24 hours, 7 days a week	Provides 24 hour rehabilitation on an inpatient basis with a maximum LoS of 31 days.
ACCESS TO THE SERVICE	Through referral to consultant physicians with an interest in the elderly.	Social Services are the referring agent based on community care criteria. The Consultant Medical Team must agree the patient is medically ready for discharge. The patient is assessed by a member of the multi-disciplinary team prior to admission.
CARE OFFERED	Multi-disciplinary assessment, plan of care, evaluation and preparation of complex discharge packages involving health and social care.	Multi professional rehabilitation therapy ranging from psychological skills development to general physio/OT
TIME LIMITATION	No – varies from a few days to several weeks	Maximum of 31 days.
RESPONSIBILITY FOR DISCHARGE	Consultant physician in consultation with multidisciplinary team.	Social services although the discharge plan is by multi agency agreement – every patient has a discharge case conference.
NO. USING SERVICE	15	28
NO. OVER PREVIOUS MONTH	38	
AGE RANGE	65+. Average age is 83 years	18-100+
TEAM MEMBERS	Nursing: 2.00 F grade, 3.00 E grade, 6.88 D grade, 11.35 A grade. Physio 0.50. OT 0.50. Social Workers. NB. This establishment also supports an eight bedded specialist woundcare unit within the same ward. Access to speech therapy, chiropody etc.	8 x Registered Nurses; 10 x CSW; 3 x Ward Assistants; 0.5 x clerk; 0.5 x OT; 0.5 x Physio; 1.0 x volunteer.
MEASURED BY/EVALUATION	A detailed ongoing evaluation is in place which considers patient/carer experience, efficiency, effective delivery, fair access, health improvements and outcomes.	LoS is a regular monitored indicator. Patient achievement against plan is measured and evaluated on an ongoing basis. Readmission rates are evaluated.
IMPACT/OUTCOMES	Reduced delays in discharge. Improved discharge planning. Extremely high patient/carer satisfaction. (recent survey showed 96% of returners as satisfied) Improved links between health and social services.	Improved patient satisfaction. Reduced readmission rates. All patients appear to improve or maintain their physical or mental status during their stay.
LESSONS LEARNT/PLANS	To consider more flexible access/referral routes and 'GP' beds. To conduct a detailed study identifying gaps in service provision which prevent a proportion of this 'vulnerable' patient groups returning to their own homes	Communication and awareness training – never too much. Plan to develop a respite service and to develop a rehabilitation day service.
DOCUMENTATION AVAILABLE	Patient/carer satisfaction questionnaire. Summary report	
CONTACT	Sandra Dixon, Senior Sister, Hawthorne Ward, Tickhill Road Hospital, Tickhill Road, Balby, Doncaster Tel: 01302 796405	Mrs M Greer, Acting Head of Nursing, George Eliot Hosp NHS Trust, College Street, Nuneaton, Warwickshire CV10 8DJ Tel: 01203 865146 Fax: 01203 865086

Social services led

NAME OF NHS TRUST	SANDWELL SOCIAL SERVICES DEPARTMENT, TIPTON CARE ORGANISATION, SANDWELL HEALTH CARE TRUST	COMMUNITY HEALTH SHEFFIELD AND SHEFFIELD SOCIAL SERVICES
NAME OF PROJECT/SCHEME	Intermediate nursing beds. Intermediate home care. Rehab daycare/residential & personal care service.	Assessment and Integrated Care Service (AICS) - previously known as Diversion of Admission Scheme.
PURPOSE OF SCHEME	Discharge at the right time, with the right package of care. Preventing admission. Encouraging rehabilitation.	To relieve pressure on hospital beds by discharging elderly patients home with a 'package' of care who would otherwise need a hospital bed – patients who are frail and elderly and have had a fall and patients with COPD.
MULTI-AGENCY INVOLVEMENT	Sandwell Social Services Department, Tipton Care Organisation, Sandwell Health Care Trust, plus providers of all involved.	Intensive Home Nursing Service, Social Services, Community Therapy Services, City Wide Alarms, Sheffield Churches Council for Community Care (SCCCC).
START DATE	3-4 years ago with progressive service development.	Winter 1997
FUNDING	From Sandwell Social Services Department, Tipton Care Organisation, Sandwell Health Care Trust, plus winter pressures funding and waiting list initiatives.	Initially – 'Winter Bed Initiative' money, then recurring health and social services funds
REASON FOR INTRODUCTION	To facilitate joint working between health and social services. To improve multidisciplinary assess. of patients	To relieve the pressure on hospital beds
LOCATION	Spot purchased beds in nursing homes and home care	Home based
AVAILABILITY OF SERVICE	Variable	9.00 to 22.00 Mon-Fri and 11.00 to 17.00 Sat-Sun. 7 days a week
ACCESS TO THE SERVICE	Via community care assessment	Patients assessed in A&E departments and if medically stable referred to AICS.
CARE OFFERED	Domiciliary through to nursing home	Appropriate care from Rapid Response Home Care Service, Intensive Home Nursing Service, City wide alarm service to support patient at home, with physiotherapy and occupational therapy services if required.
TIME LIMITATION	No time limit	Free for 7 days.
RESPONSIBILITY FOR DISCHARGE	Care Manager	Social worker reassesses. After 7 days patients may be referred to mainstream services.
TEAM MEMBERS	3 community nurses x 1.0; 2 clerical assistants x 1.0; social services input - 1 hospital social work practitioner x 0.4.	1 x scheme manager; 5 x assessment team; 1.25 x clerical officer; 1.60 x occupational therapists; 1.30 x physiotherapists; 0.3 x consultant geriatrician; 1.0 x Falls Clinic nurse; 2.0 x B grade auxiliaries; 0.5 x SCCCC Co-ordinator.
MEASURED BY/EVALUATION	Process and outcomes are being measured	SCCCC - Patient questionnaire.
IMPACT/OUTCOMES	Improvement in general health; promotion of care in primary settings	During pilot scheme, 8th December 1997-31st March 1998, 1858 bed nights were saved with 293 cases. This equates to 16 hospital beds saved.
LESSONS LEARNT/PLANS	More integration reduces duplication, achieves better assessments – use of resources and improved outcomes	To continue with the scheme if funding obtained.
DOCUMENTATION AVAILABLE	Service outline and access criteria. Service leaflet	
CONTACT	Paul Charnock, Locality Commissioning Manager, North West Adult Care Team, Sandwell Social Service Department, 6 Stockdale Parade, Tipton, West Midlands DY4 8QL Tel: 0121 569 5953	Helen Clark, Co-ordinator Intensive Home Nursing Service, Woodhouse Clinic, 3 Skelton Lane, Sheffield, S13 7LY Tel: 0114-254 8760 Fax: 0114-269 1916

Social services led

WIGAN SOCIAL SERVICES DEPARTMENT. WIGAN & BOLTON HA, WIGAN & LEIGH NHS TRUST	*NAME OF NHS TRUST*	**BRISTOL SOCIAL SERVICES, UNITED BRISTOL HEALTHCARE TRUST**
Ambleside Bank Older Persons Resource Centre	*NAME OF PROJECT/SCHEME*	South Bristol Rehabilitation Centre
To provide Resource Centre for older people, including residential multidisc. assessment, follow-up day & respite care, based on Helen Hamlyn Foundations Epics	*PURPOSE OF SCHEME*	To provide social rehabilitation for older people to enable them to remain within their own homes
ALM Medical Services Ltd (independent sector) own and staff the purpose built centre. Trust employed OT's and physiotherapists, and social worker	*MULTI-AGENCY INVOLVEMENT*	Social Service/Health
March 1996	*START DATE*	Oct 98 - 7 beds, April 99 - 12 beds, April 2000 - 20 beds
Social Services block contract for 80% of the places and Spot Purchase the remainder. They employ Social Worker. Joint finance used for OT's/physios employed by Trust	*FUNDING*	Social Services capital investment for 3 years
To prevent admissions to residential care for the most vulnerable people, eg. on discharge from hospital.To assist in maintaining older people in their own homes	*REASON FOR INTRODUCTION*	To provide wider range of options/facilities for older people to enable them to remain in own homes and prevent unnecessary admissions to residential care
Social services	*LEAD CLINICIAN*	Social services manager with OT/Physiotherapist support
Single residential home. A second assessment centre providing nursing care is planned	*LOCATION*	Rehabilitation Centre
24 hours, 7 days a week	*AVAILABILITY OF SERVICE*	24 hours, 7 days a week
Following a social work assessment, the manager and social worker decide on admission. OT and physio assessment can assist the decision	*ACCESS TO THE SERVICE*	Referrals made from a range of professionals including Social Workers, Occupational Therapists, Physiotherapists, GPs, Nurses etc.
Residential assessment; day care; residential respite care; support to carers; information.	*CARE OFFERED*	OT and Physio draw up individual rehabilitation programmes which service users follow with the help of Care Officers who also provide hands-on care as necessary. Medical input provided by GPs and DNs
Initial assessment minimum 2 to maximum 12 weeks. Day care and programmed respite care ongoing	*TIME LIMITATION*	No longer than 8 weeks, usually 4-6
A care planning meeting chaired by the social worker	*RESPONSIBILITY FOR DISCHARGE*	Centre Manager (Social Services Manager)
30 Residential. 10 Day Care	*NO. USING SERVICE*	October 1998 – 7 beds
January = 24. Av pm over past 14 months = 31	*NO. OVER PREVIOUS MONTH*	7 in March 1999
65+	*AGE RANGE*	65-95
Care staff employed by ALM Medical Services Ltd. 1 Senior OT, 1 Junior OT. 1 Senior Physiotherapist, 2 OT part time assistants, 1 Social Worker	*TEAM MEMBERS*	1 Centre Manager, 2 Assistant Centre Managers, 5.3 Care Officers, 2 Night Care Assistants, 0.5 Admin Assistant, 2.7 Domestics, 1 Cook. 1 OT and 1 Physio
Statistics collected to monitor admissions and discharges. Small research project undertaken to consider outcomes for individuals.	*MEASURED BY/EVALUATION*	Too early for measured outcomes yet. Full evaluation of first year in October 1999. Also measuring services needed after discharge compared with readmission.
70% of people admitted return to their own homes. 56% of people admitted from hospital return to own homes – at high risk of being admitted to residential care.	*IMPACT/OUTCOMES*	Referrals increasing weekly as professionals use the services. Need to be in operation for full year to evaluate full impact.
The Centre has not admitted as many people as expected from hospital (22%), possibly due to the high level of care needs- 2nd Centre planned. Linked to whole system approach to preventing admissions to hospital, facilitating discharge and maintaining people in the community.	*LESSONS LEARNT/PLANS*	
Information on Epics and Helen Hamlyn foundation. Specification for Centre.	*DOCUMENTATION AVAILABLE*	Issues paper for future due in May 1999. Leaflet describing service offered. Brochure under preparation.
Barbara Hitchins, Service Manager, Wigan SS Dept, Nurses' Home 3, Billinge Hospital, Upholland Road, Billinge, Wigan, WN5 7ET Tel: 01695 626464 Eve Crabtree, Ass. Dir. of Commiss, Wigan & Leigh NHS Trust, Bryan House, Standishgate, Wigan Tel: 01942 244000	*CONTACT*	Nikki Cole, Team Manager, Welsman, Bishop Street, St Pauls, Bristol, BS2 9JA Tel: 0117-9036734 Fax: 0117 9036739; Sue Moore, Centre Manager, SBRC, c/o Woodcroft, 30 Inns Court Green, Knowle, Bristol BS4 1TF Tel: 0117 9530754

Other approaches

NAME OF NHS TRUST	HALTON GENERAL HOSPITAL NHS TRUST, RUNCORN	NORTH STAFFORDSHIRE COMBINED HEALTHCARE NHS TRUST - COMMUNITY TRUST
NAME OF PROJECT/SCHEME	Rapid Response Respiratory Team	Residential Rehabilitation for older clients in Stone
PURPOSE OF SCHEME	Prevent admission to hospital. Facilitate early discharge	To enable quicker, co-ordinated discharge from hospital for clients needing rehabiliation prior to returning home, to offer short-term rehab and faciltate change in use of nursing home respite beds.
MULTI-AGENCY INVOLVEMENT	Rapid response respiratory team (including consultant physician, specialist respiratory nurse, respiratory physiotherapist, staff nurse and nurse auxiliary), district nursing service from community trust, local GPs.	Health and social services, GPs and private nursing home.
START DATE	December 1997	Evolved from existing Health Respite Beds.
FUNDING	Initially 'Winter pressure' funding 97/98, but continued by local HA possibly for consolidated funding 1999/2000	Funding bid was not successful, so project now within resources plus bed from Social Services.
REASON FOR INTRODUCTION	33% of Halton Hospital medical emergencies are result of respiratory illness. Higher than national av. chronic chest problems, 5th highest for lung cancer in the country	Identified need by rehab team, GPs and social services. Natural development of use of respite beds.
LEAD CLINICIAN	Lead clinician- consultant. GP retains medical responsibility for patient in community	
LOCATION	Own home, residential/nursing homes.	Nursing home and rehab centre
AVAILABILITY OF SERVICE	24 hours, 7 days a week. New referrals only taken between 9.00-17.00 Mon-Fri	Beds - 24 hours, 7 days a week. Rehab staff - 5 days (9.00 - 17.00), but open to review.
ACCESS TO THE SERVICE	Via direct line to service – 24 hours a day. GP referral, hospital doctors/ hospital bed manager	By referral to Stone Rehabilitation Service (SRS).
CARE OFFERED	Acute mgt. of respiratory illness. Intensive home care. Nurse/physio led clinics (medical support by staff grade doctor). Nebulizer service. Pulmonary rehab programme.	24 hour nursing care and GP cover. Rehabilitation goals. Maintenance goals. Rehabilitation review.
TIME LIMITATION	No	6 weeks
RESPONSIBILITY FOR DISCHARGE	Nurse/physio in consultation with patient's GP	Stone Rehab Service and GPs.
NO. USING SERVICE	Max 54 (although at height of winter were seeing 80)	
NO. OVER PREVIOUS MONTH	38 new referrals	
AGE RANGE	Average age is 71, ranging 30-80+	65+ but may be extended to include under 65s.
TEAM MEMBERS	Consultant lead x 1;grade H respiratory nurse specialist x 1; hospital nurse specialist; Sen I specialist respiratory physiotherapis; staff nurse grade E x 1; auxiliary nurse grade A x 1; admin and clerical support x 1.	2 x physiotherapists; 2 x occupational therapists; 0.5 x speech therapists; 0.2 x chiropody; 0.6 x research co-ordinator; 4.8 x rehab assistants; 1.3 x admin; 0.4 x support services.
MEASURED BY/EVALUATION	GP satisfaction survey. Reduced LOS for respiratory patients. Readmission rates for respiratory illness down. Reduced number of patients admitted with respiratory illness. DoH evaluation of project.	Cost savings; qualitative evaluations (user and staff questionnaires and interviews).
IMPACT/OUTCOMES	313 patients seen and cared for. Only 36 went on to require admission to hospital out of 209 GP referrals. GPs said all 209 referrals would have been admitted if service had not been available. Presented at winter BTS meeting. Presenting at American TS meeting - April 1999	Accessing team via one referral. Early intervention work leading to prevention of unnecessary hospital admission. Rehab review beds have clarified difference between health/social respite beds.
LESSONS LEARNT/PLANS	Consolidated funding. Roll-out to Warrington with second team. BiPAP (Non-invasive positive pressure ventilation) to be available in patient's own home	See description of SRS in 'Directory of Developments' (1998) NHS Executive. Article by Shield F (1998) 2. Developing a therapy-led community rehabilitation team. *Managing Community Care*, Vol 6, Issue 4, pp 160-168.
CONTACT	Bev Critchlow, General Clinical Manager, Adult Medicine, Halton General Hospital NHS Trust, Runcorn, Cheshire WA7 3DA Tel: 01928 753373	Fiona Shield, Stone Rehabilitation Service, Stafford Road, Stone, Staffordshire ST15 0ME Tel: 01785 813311 Fax: 01785 811334 e-mail: stonerehab@btinternet.com

Other approaches

CAMDEN AND ISLINGTON COMMUNITY HEALTH NHS TRUST	NAME OF NHS TRUST	CAMDEN AND ISLINGTON COMMUNITY HEALTH NHS TRUST
The Community Rehabilitation Team	NAME OF PROJECT/SCHEME	Nursing and Therapy Support Team to statutory and private residential and nursing homes in Camden and Islington
Provides assessment, advice, therapy and support for people who have multiple physical and neurological disabilities	PURPOSE OF SCHEME	To provide nursing and therapy advice and support for enabling residents to retain their independence within the residential setting, thus avoiding transfer to a nursing home. Assist primary care services to enable elderly people, particularly recently discharged from hospital, to live in residential settings. Provide advice/support for residential and nursing home staff in the management of the health needs of residents.
Multidisciplinary service: medical, speech and language, occupational and physiotherapy, clinical psychology	MULTI-AGENCY INVOLVEMENT	Community Trust. Royal Free Hospital Trust. Camden and Islington Health Authority. London Borough of Camden. London Borough of Islington.
April 1998	START DATE	October 1998
Health Authority	FUNDING	Whole System bid for 6 months. £104,000.00
Health Authority revised Physical Disability Service. Proposed to de-commission a Medical Rehabilitation Service and re-commission a Community Rehab Team	REASON FOR INTRODUCTION	Increase in frail elderly population in R&N Homes with increased demand for health advice and support. Prevent unnecessary admission of hospital or transfer from residential to nursing home. Access to specialist advice
Team Leader - Consultant in Community Rehabilitation	LEAD CLINICIAN	Team co-managed by G grade nurse and senior occupational therapist
Community centre and patients' homes	LOCATION	Residential homes
9.00 to 17.00 Monday to Friday	AVAILABILITY OF SERVICE	9.00 to 17.00. Monday to Friday
Via written/telephone referral. Referrals accepted from: GPs and PCTs, hospital based clinicians, A&E, LA Care Management, OTs. Also self-referrals (if known to service) and key-workers.	ACCESS TO THE SERVICE	Each Team member is link person to named Home and attends Home for referrals, team meetings. Referrals can be faxed, written to team office at St Pancras.
Generic assessment and specific uni-disciplinary assessments. Seamless access into treatment programme from in-patients following discharge. A mix of Centre and home-based treatment . Advice on disability management, and Care Packages.	CARE OFFERED	Initial audit of homes. Specific assessment including nursing and therapy. Generic assessments including risk assessments. Specific training programme for care workers. Links to acute units regarding admission and discharges.
The team leader and relevant senior clinicians	RESPONSIBILITY FOR DISCHARGE	The team
125 patients currently. 20 awaiting assessment School leavers to late sixties. Some older patients referred to older people's services	NO. USING SERVICE AGE RANGE	Frail elderly.
1x consultant; 1x clinical psychologist; 1x Head III physiotherapist (clinical specialist); 1x Senior II physiotherapist (rotational post); 1x Senior speech and language therapist; 1x Head III OT; 1x Senior I OT; 1x Basic Grade OT (rotational), 1x A&CH; 0.50 x A&C3.	TEAM MEMBERS	1x G grade nurse; 2x F grade nurses; 0.80 x Sen occupational therapist; 0.50 x Sen physiotherapist. Advice from consultant physician and clinical services manager for nursing.
Team has not had any formal evaluations to date. Produces statistics for Trust and HA. Regular contact meeting with HA.	MEASURED BY/EVALUATION	Half-way & final report. Use of standardised assessment documentation. Analysis of referrals and their outcome. Analysis of training outcome.
Audit Programme agreed. Team undertaking 3 projects: looking at team interventions for stroke, head injuries, school leavers.Service plan includes closer links between Team and Care Management, supporting development of Centre for Independent Living.	IMPACT/PLANS	
Dr Steven Luttrell, Team Leader CRT, Peckwater Centre, 6 Peckwater Street, London NW5 2TX Tel: 0171-530 6400	CONTACT	Jan Joseph, Clinical Services Manager, Kentish Town Health Centre, Bartholomew Road London NW5 Tel: 0171-530 4700

Other approaches

MILTON KEYNES GENERAL HOSPITAL TRUST	NAME OF NHS TRUST	NEWCASTLE CITY HEALTH TRUST. NEWCASTLE HOUSING DEPARTMENT (LOCAL AUTHORITY)
Pulmonary Rehabilitation Programme	NAME OF PROJECT/SCHEME	Nurse led units in 'Shieldfield Sheltered Housing Scheme'
Improved exercise capacity and quality of life. Reduced in-patient admissions	PURPOSE OF SCHEME	To prevent patients over 60 years being admitted to hospital by timely therapeutic nursing intervention.
Occupational therapy, dietetics, respiratory nurse, social worker, respiratory physician, physiotherapist	MULTI-AGENCY INVOLVEMENT	Health, housing, social services and user group of older people. (Action for Health Older People Newcastle.)
January 1998	START DATE	August 1998
Whole Systems funding	FUNDING	Health authority (Newcastle and North Tyne). Housing (Capital) Department – City Council.
Pressure on emergency services	REASON FOR INTRODUCTION	To provide a local unit where older people or carers could have therapeutic care which prevents them from being admitted to an acute hospital.
Senior I Physiotherapist – overall co-ordination and planning. Chest Physician – oversees clinical issues	LEAD CLINICIAN	District nurse
Physio gym, Milton Keynes General	LOCATION	In a sheltered housing scheme
Per patient = 4 hours/week for 6 weeks	AVAILABILITY OF SERVICE	24 hours, 7 days a week
Via GP referral and hospital consultant	ACCESS TO THE SERVICE	Via patient's district nurse
Programme of exercise and education	CARE OFFERED	Intensive therapeutic nursing, carers support, respite care, education and training for patients or carers.
6 week programme	TIME LIMITATION	14 days
Senior I Physiotherapist	RESPONSIBILITY FOR DISCHARGE	District nurse
4-5	NO. USING SERVICE	4
12	NO. OVER PREVIOUS MONTH	
35-75	AGE RANGE	Over 60
Senior I Physio 21 hours, OT 3 hours, Dietician 1/2 hour, Respiratory Nurse 1 hours, Physio helper 2 hours, Social worker 1 hour/week	TEAM MEMBERS	G grade district nurse x 1. B grade support workers.
St George's respiratory questionnaire. Hospital anxiety and depression scale. 10 metre shuttle walk test.	MEASURED BY/EVALUATION	Evaluation by Senior Research Nurse, Newcastle General Hospital.
Currently being collated by Clinical Effectiveness Unit	IMPACT/OUTCOMES	User group involved in 'Action for Health Older People' Ppoject team leading to new relationships formed between health, housing and social services. Partnership working between local housing officers and health workers. Strategic partnership: Housing Directorate, Health Authority and Newcastle City Trust.
Establishing support groups with Breathe Easy. Closer interaction with GP practices	LESSONS LEARNT/PLANS	Early stage uncertainty among some groups of professionals which is being addressed.
	DOCUMENTATION AVAILABLE	Information leaflets for press and patients.
Ms Bernadette Dunne Tel: 01908 660033 bleep 1338	CONTACT	Yvonne Birkett, Assistant General Manager (East Locality), Ravenswood Clinic, Ravenswood Road, Newcastle upon Tyne, Tel: 0191-219 4641

Other approaches

SOUTH WEST LONDON COMMUNITY TRUST	*NAME OF NHS TRUST*	BEDFORDSHIRE AND LUTON COMMUNITY TRUST
Domiciliary Physiotherapy Service for Adults	*NAME OF PROJECT/SCHEME*	Acquired Brain Injury (ABI) Team
Facilitate early discharge, and prevent admission to hospital	*PURPOSE OF SCHEME*	To case manage patients with acquired brain injury and complex needs
Intermediate care nurse practitioner, day care unit	*MULTI-AGENCY INVOLVEMENT*	Social Services, primary and acute health services, Headway, specialist services.
In place for several years	*START DATE*	September 1997
Health Authorities	*FUNDING*	Recurrent funding secured.
Initially to manage respiratory patients at home and try to keep them out of hospital	*REASON FOR INTRODUCTION*	Lack of coordination across continuum of care. Lack of specialist clinical input and reviews for patients on continuing care. Belief that continuing care and block contract resources could be managed better.
Physiotherapist	*LEAD CLINICIAN*	Different clinicians (OT, Psychologist) take lead on different cases according to clinical needs of the patient.
Care provided in patients homes	*LOCATION*	Team will see patients wherever they are located.
8.00 - 17.00, Monday to Friday	*AVAILABILITY OF SERVICE*	Mainly 9.00 - 17.00 with some flexibility, 5 days a week.
Referral from GPs, hospital consultants and other therapists, acute primary nurse practitioner, district nurse, HVs and social services.	*ACCESS TO THE SERVICE*	Open referral system. Typically referrals will come from acute hospital or social services.
Physiotherapy for patients with acute chest problems, acute back pain, chronic CVA, post operative orthopaedic surgery, treatment for frail elderly.	*CARE OFFERED*	Assessment, case management and collaboration to guide other services.
Average episode ranges from 3-6 visits. Can provide longer episodes of care.	*TIME LIMITATION*	No
Physiotherapist	*RESPONSIBILITY FOR DISCHARGE*	
3460 contacts for 1998	*NO. USING SERVICE*	65
3460 contacts for 1998	*NO. OVER PREVIOUS MONTH*	
18 years +	*AGE RANGE*	19-74 at present, but age range is not restricted.
3.4 x Senior I PT, 1.0 x Senior II PT, 0.42 x Assistant	*TEAM MEMBERS*	Consultant Clinical Psychologist x0.5; 2 Clinical Coordinator - Head III OT x1.6 2 Assistant Psychologists x 1.1
Patient satisfaction surveys to check meeting of Patient Charter and local standards	*MEASURED BY/EVALUATION*	Basic screening re impairment, disability. User views determined informally. Achievement of set goals. Adherence to agreed care plan.
Highly valued by GPs	*IMPACT/OUTCOMES*	Regular monitoring of clinical needs. Care pathway streamlined. More patient focused care plans.
Need to extend service	*LESSONS LEARNT/PLANS*	Need an ABI community treatment service. Research into outcome measurement for ABI rehab. Aim is to compare effectiveness of inpatient and community based programmes.
Service protocol	*DOCUMENTATION AVAILABLE*	Report describing team is available but is being updated to reflect the evolving roles within the team.
Josephine Jackson, Superintendent Physiotherapist, Putney Hospital Tel: 0181 789 6633	*CONTACT*	Helen Badge, Clinical Coordinator, ABI Team, Intermediate Care Services, Disability Resource Centre, Poynters Road, Dunstable LU5 4TP Tel: 01582 709021 Fax: 01582 709057

Other approaches

FIRST COMMUNITY NHS TRUST	*NAME OF NHS TRUST*	NEWCASTLE CITY HEALTH NHS TRUST (COMMUNITY REHABILITATION TRUST)
Great Wyrley Reablement Service	*NAME OF PROJECT/SCHEME*	Stroke Discharge Team
To reduce admission to residential care and dependency on community services	*PURPOSE OF SCHEME*	To facilitate early discharge of stroke patients
Health - Occupational and physiotherapy Social Services - Social workers, community care workers	*MULTI-AGENCY INVOLVEMENT*	Social Worker is part of team but otherwise all from same Trust
October 1998	*START DATE*	February 1995
Social Services Challenge fund	*FUNDING*	Health Authority
Unacceptably high demand for residential placements direct from hospital	*REASON FOR INTRODUCTION*	High demand on acute medical beds, cost of stroke patients to NHS. Team set up as part of Research project.
No lead clinician	*LEAD CLINICIAN*	Co-ordinators of team - OT/PT Job-share
Residential and home care	*LOCATION*	At home
24 hours, 7 days a week	*AVAILABILITY OF SERVICE*	Variable according to care package or therapy.
Via social worker	*ACCESS TO THE SERVICE*	By anyone in hospital setting but would need doctor's agreement for early discharge.
In-patient and community reablement	*CARE OFFERED*	Home care is available from the team to suit needs of patient/carer. OT, PT, SaLT, SW all available for ongoing treatment.
Up to 13 weeks	*TIME LIMITATION*	Depends on patient achieving goals.
The whole team	*RESPONSIBILITY FOR DISCHARGE*	The team with the guidance of Co-ordinator
4 in-patients (to be increased); up to 20 comm. clients	*NO. USING SERVICE*	Current caseload 30-40 patients
12	*NO. OVER PREVIOUS MONTH*	New referrals - 12
Mainly 65+	*AGE RANGE*	Any adult
0.5 senior OT (to be increased to 1.0), 0.4 senior physio (may also be increased to 1.0)	*TEAM MEMBERS*	Co-ordinator OP/PT Job-share 1.0, OT Senior I x 1.75, PT Senior Ix 2.00, SW x 0.5, SALT x 0.7 Assistant x 1.0, Technician x 0.5, Admin/clerical x 1.0
TELER, Community Dependency Index, Goal achievement	*MEASURED BY/EVALUATION*	Initially evaluated by Randomised Controlled Trial. Currently being evaluated by Stroke Association over 3 year period.
Too early to measure impact objectively. All but one clients have gone home or remained there	*IMPACT/OUTCOMES*	Service now integrated into city-wide strategy. Patients supported home early from Acute Trust, Stroke Unit and Elderly Care beds. Currently about 150 patients a year.
More interagency training required	*LESSONS LEARNT/PLANS*	Looking at extending service to address other stroke patients needs not just acute admission/discharge.
Service protocols, Samples of client records	*DOCUMENTATION AVAILABLE*	Papers published in Clinical Rehabilitation following research. Listed in directory of Developments – NHS Executive.
D. Martin, Senior Occupational Therapist, Great Wyrley Reablement Service, 156 Walsall Road, Great Wyrley, Walsall Tel: 01922 410983	*CONTACT*	Jackie Moon/Barbara Tait, Service Co-ordinators, Stroke Discharge Team, St Nicholas Hospital, Jubilee Road, Newcastle upon Tyne NE3 3XT Tel/fax: 0191-223 2219

Other approaches

NAME OF NHS TRUST	**THE SOUTH BUCKINGHAMSHIRE NHS TRUST (ACUTE AND COMMUNITY)**
NAME OF PROJECT/SCHEME	EPICS – Elderly Persons Integrated Care System
PURPOSE OF SCHEME	To maintain people over 65 in the community by co-ordinating flexible, responsive packages of care according to assessed needs; to facilitate earlier discharge
MULTI-AGENCY INVOLVEMENT	Social services, GPs, OTs, physios, hospital staff, voluntary organisations and local communities.
START DATE	Marlow, April 1994; Bourne End, Dec. 1996; Chesham/ Amersham, November 1998; High Wycombe, May 1999
FUNDING	Pilot project in Marlow funded by Joint Finance initially. Joint Finance is funding the Managed Intranet pilot over 3 years. Now Joint Finance, Winter Funding and Whole Systems Initiatives to reduce Waiting Lists. Projects supported by local commercial companies and Charities
LEAD CLINICIAN	Consultant Physician in General Medicine as advisor
LOCATION	Hospitals and community
AVAILABILITY OF SERVICE	9.00 to 17.00 weekdays. (Weekends and bank holidays via mobile phone). Out of hours 17.00 - 21.00 via community hospital. Care workers 8.00 to 22.00
ACCESS TO THE SERVICE	Through DNs, community hospital or care workers
CARE OFFERED	Provision of information and guidance (resources database). Home assessment visit of EPICS Co-ordinator. Co-ordination of immediate care plan involving other providers, volunteers etc. Multidisciplinary assessment; care worker in the home; EPICS Phone Link
TIME LIMITATION	2 weeks
RESPONSIBILITY FOR DISCHARGE	The EPICS Co-ordinator
NO. USING SERVICE	Marlow only: Approx 16 (285 referrals in 1998).
NO. OVER PREVIOUS MONTH	Marlow only: 32 (new referrals)
AGE RANGE	Average age 86
TEAM MEMBERS	Development Manager Managerial scale 24, 3 Co-ordinators G grade nurse (or equivalent) (1 per site), assisted by 3 Care Worker organisers (1 per site) (18 hours) F grade nurse (or equivalent). Administrative Officers (1FTE per site) A&C grade 4 Chesham and Wycombe sites, Clerical and Data Assistants (1 FTE) A&C grade 3 Marlow site, Data Supervisor (15 hours) A&C grade 5. Voluntary Team Leaders for Phone Link. EPICS Care Workers B grade nurse equivalent.
MEASURED BY/EVALUATION	An Evaluation Report (1997) with audit of admissions; user satis. survey using critical incident technique; practitioner satisfaction. Annual Review.
IMPACT/OUTCOMES	Bed day and efficiency savings as demonstrated by Audit. Effective for users and professionals - surveys. Benefits to SS - time gained for assess. & shared care. Develop. of series of implementation models that can be flexibly transposed & set of new values for Integrated Care
DOCUMENTATION AVAILABLE	EPICS – New Ways with Old Services. Evaluation of Marlow EPICS. Audrey Calviou 1997
CONTACT	Margaret Allen, Development Manager, c/o EPICS, Chesham Community Hospital Hospital Hill, Waterside, Chesham Bucks HP5 1PJ Tel: 07979 770261 Fax: 01494 783554